PANDORA'S CLOCK

Maureen Freely was born in New Jersey, grew up in Istanbul, and now lives in Bath. She has a degree from Harvard University and has published three novels: *Mother's Helper*, *The Life of the Party* and *The Stork Club*. Her columns, book reviews, essays and features have appeared in the *Independent on Sunday*, the *Observer*, the *Guardian*, the *New Statesman and Society*, *Cosmopolitan*, *Options*, *Woman's Journal*, *Women's Review*, and *Marxism Today*. She has four children – 57% of whom were planned – and two stepchildren.

Celia Pyper is a General Practitioner in Oxford, having qualified from London University, and also has an Oxford Certificate in Psychotherapy. She is a Tutor in General Practice at Oxford University. Her practice has a specialist interest in teaching fertility awareness. She has presented research on the subject in Washington, D.C., Nairobi, and in many teaching hospitals in Britain. At present she is doing Family Planning Research in the Department of Public Health and Primary Care at Oxford University. She is active in promoting health education and preventative medicine in schools and colleges as well as in General Practice. She is married with three children.

Other titles by the authors

MAUREEN FREELY

Fiction
**Mother's Helper
The Life of the Party
The Stork Club**

PANDORA'S CLOCK

Understanding our Fertility

*The choices we face over
contraception, pregnancy, genetic screening,
abortion and infertility*

MAUREEN FREELY and CELIA PYPER

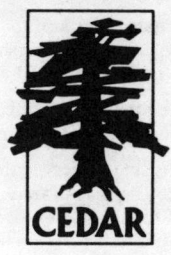

A Mandarin Paperback
PANDORA'S CLOCK

First published in Great Britain 1993
by William Heinemann Ltd
This edition published 1994
by Mandarin Paperbacks
an imprint of Reed Consumer Books Ltd
Michelin House, 81 Fulham Road, London SW3 6RB
and Auckland, Melbourne, Singapore and Toronto

Copyright © Maureen Freely and Celia Pyper 1993
The authors have asserted their moral rights

A CIP catalogue record for this title
is available from the British Library
ISBN 0 7493 1987 9

Printed and bound in Great Britain by
Cox & Wyman Ltd, Reading, Berks

This book is sold subject to the condition
that it shall not, by way of trade or otherwise,
be lent, resold, hired out, or otherwise circulated
without the publisher's prior consent in any form
of binding or cover other than that in which
it is published and without a similar condition
including this condition being imposed
on the subsequent purchaser.

ACKNOWLEDGEMENTS

We would like to thank Toni Belfield and Joan Walsh of the Family Planning Association for their helpful advice and up to date information, Dr Elizabeth Clubb and Jane Knight for their advice on fertility awareness, Dr Elizabeth Greenhall for her advice on family planning, Mr Steven Kennedy for his help on infertility investigations, Sally Dakin and Shona Reed-Purvis for information on health education and risk-taking, Jill Thomas for her very useful general comments, the National Women's Register and Bill Heine of Radio Oxford for helping us launch our research, Marianne Stanley for being there, Polly Spearman for looking after all those children, and Dr John Clubb for his tireless computer support, always supplied with a tactful smile and an undeserved cup of coffee.

To Ben, Frank, and all their children

CONTENTS

PREFACE	Why Did We Decide To Write This Book?	xi
ONE	Anatomy of a Rational Decision	1
TWO	The Wanted Child, the Prepared Parent and the Double Standard	9
THREE	Wishes, Plans and Excuses	15
FOUR	Imperfect Understandings	27
FIVE	Who Controls the Means of Reproduction?	35
SIX	Hiccups and Surprises	43
SEVEN	Whose Decision Is It Anyway?	53
EIGHT	The Final Solution	75
NINE	When Nature Has the Last Laugh: Unplanned Infertility	81
TEN	What Is Wrong With This Picture?	97
ELEVEN	The Trouble With Doctors	103
TWELVE	A Beautiful Picture	109
THIRTEEN	Fertility is Political	127
FOURTEEN	The Downgraded Parent, the Perfectible Child and the Spectre of Eugenics	143
FIFTEEN	How Fertile Are We?	153
SIXTEEN	Fertility Control: the Choices on Offer	165
SEVENTEEN	How Serious Is the Threat of Infertility	211
EIGHTEEN	And Finally – There's No Such Thing as a Mistake	231
	Appendices	239
	Glossary	241
	Notes	251
	Bibliography	255
	Useful Addresses	260
	Index	269

PREFACE

WHY DID WE DECIDE TO WRITE THIS BOOK?

It began as a conversational brain teaser. We had long been aware of a wide and puzzling gap between the way people talked about family planning in public and the stories to which they admitted in private. In the official versions, contraception was a cinch, children were planned and wanted, and decisions joint. In the versions people told when they could be sure their story would never go beyond the walls of a surgery or the ears of a friend, meanwhile, there were all the dramas and passions of grand opera. Even where the results *looked* happy, people spoke of terrible inner struggles, unforgivable betrayals, irrational fears, frustrated desires, uncontrollable guilt, and wrecked lives.

How to explain this discrepancy? And what to make of the tiny roles given in almost all these stories to the facts of life? Despite the fact that a good number of their authors had had the benefit of sex education, their understanding of fertility was often narrow and patchy. Few, for example, had the faintest idea how long a woman was likely to be fertile during a given cycle, while many were governed by a nightmarish image they dared not examine too closely called the biological clock. Why such fear and ignorance in an age that was meant to be so enlightened about sex? We decided to find out.

How do people *really* plan their children? When we looked at the professional literature generated by social scientists, family planning agencies and the medical professions, the focus (with a few honourable exceptions) was on 'problem groups' – teenagers who didn't use contraception, women in developing countries who had too many children for their own good, the mysterious and ever growing battalions of women in the developed world who used abortion as their preferred method of birth control, and the distraught couples who presented themselves for fertility treatment. We found all these topics to be popular in the media, too, along with an insatiable interest in 'new' types of parenting – women who had babies 'artificially', or alone, or late, or with a lesbian partner; men who were primary, or equal, caretakers. These scenarios often provided opportunities for the writer to discuss what ought and ought not to be the prerequisites of parenthood.

It was a huge job, everyone agreed. It involved unspeakable sacrifices and so was not to be entered into lightly. If the aim in having a child was to end up with a well-adjusted, high-achieving eighteen-year-old, then everything had to go like clockwork. The birth had to be rewarding for the mother as well as safe for the child; bonding had to proceed without a hitch, breast-feeding had to continue long enough to provide immunity and nourishment but not so long as to increase the child's risk of heart disease in middle age . . . and then there was the environment to worry about. It had to be smoke- and tension-free, and full of stimulating toys, enriching activities, and confidence-building playmates. . . . One false step and all could be lost. Clearly, you had to be in A1 condition before you even entertained the possibility of parenthood. The key to success was in making sure you began at the most auspicious time. This might sound like a tall order, but almost all the literature assumed, without bothering to check for proof, that there existed beyond the twilight zone of problem groups and exceptions a sober, steady group of men and women who were as good at managing their reproductive choices as they were at negotiating their mortgages and paying into their pension plans.

So we went out to find these people and hear what they had to say. Although we began with what we thought were open minds, we found we had many assumptions to be challenged. Over the past year and a half, we have used a semi-structured interview technique to listen to both women and men, from a wide spectrum of social and

Preface

cultural backgrounds, both in this country and in the US, about how they made – or intend to make – their plans for children. Although each story is unique, we have found that while just about everyone welcomes the introduction of reproductive choice into their lives, precisely no one has had an easy time with the problems and dilemmas choice has created. There is no privileged group that has got it right. The new, improved Hobson's Multiple Choice Question looms large over all ages, classes, countries, and religions.

Set the personal dramas against the political controversies about abortion, population control, feminism, and traditional family values that are raging in the background – count the ways in which they filter into everyday life and decision-making – and the picture that emerges is of a battleground. A battleground so riddled with land mines that anyone emerging from it in one piece – let alone with a *family* – deserves the George Cross.

To do definitive studies of the problems onto which we have stumbled and the trends we have detected would take several lifetimes. And so we're not going to pretend to be speaking here as irrefutable authorities. On the other hand, the information we have gathered does beg questions about the people and agencies who have set themselves up as authorities today. We are not speaking about professionals who come into daily contact with the public, but about those higher up who conduct the studies, set the terms of the debate and shape the policies. While their intentions are almost always good, we find their terms of discussion ill-defined, their aims blinkered, and their varied prejudices unmonitored. Most appalling is their inability – or is it their unwillingness? – to respect their raw material. All too often they take the tone of the old woman who lived in a shoe and did not know what to do about her silly, headstrong dependants. 'How many times do we have to show them the light?' the professionals complain to each other. 'When *will* they ever learn?' they sigh learnedly. They do not seem to understand the strains that the current fertility debate puts on the individual. It is framed in such a way as to make even moderate success almost impossible. But we see no reason why it shouldn't be reframed, and that, in the end, is why we are writing this book: to suggest a different and more humane way of understanding fertility in general, and to provide the individual reader with the wherewithal to change Pandora's clock from an unpredictable enemy into a manageable and self-contained friend.

CHAPTER ONE

ANATOMY OF A RATIONAL DECISION

Jack and Jill have decided that the time has come to start a family. They have a house with a garden, two cars, and a healthy savings account. They have been married for four years – long enough to know it's for better rather than for worse. Jack is at a point in his career where he can afford to let the pressure off without damaging his long-term prospects. Jill, who has been working in a job she does not find fully satisfying, looks forward to taking a few years off. They plan to have two children with a gap of two years between them – although they are not averse to the idea of a third.

They decide that the best time for the first baby to arrive is the following June, not just because the weather will be better, but because they plan to visit Australia in January. If Jill conceives in September, she will be over her morning sickness by then but not so far advanced as to make a long flight dangerous.

Jill takes her last pill in the middle of August, content in the knowledge that she and her husband have made a rational decision.

That's the official version, anyway. Here's the same story with some of the background sketched in:

Jack and Jill have decided that the time is right to start a family. Or rather, Jill, who was hit with a sudden attack of broodiness on her thirty-second birthday – not long after hearing that her younger sister was pregnant with twins – has finally convinced an apprehensive and reluctant Jack that the time could not be better for her to come off the pill. After all, they have the money, don't they? Their house is worth twice what it was when they bought it. Admittedly,

I

the garden is on the small side, but then again they have every reason to move up the housing ladder. Jack's star at work is rising, and business has never been better.

As Jack does not happen to be the owner of a crystal ball, he is not to know that his prospects will look very different a year into a recession. If he is nervous about the prospect of a family, it is for emotional, rather than financial reasons. He has recently ended an unhappy affair at the office. Although it was never serious enough – at least on his part – to threaten his marriage, it has, nevertheless, made him realise that Jill and he are perhaps not ideally suited to one another. But he feels too compromised to say so when Jill first mentions her desire for children.

When Jill tells Jack she wants at least two of them, and possibly even three, he is only just able to stifle a scream. 'No,' he manages to say in a shaky voice. 'Let's take this one step at a time.' And Jill says, 'Fine.' She is not alarmed by his tone of voice because she knows men are 'just like that'. It's pregnancy that makes him nervous. Once the child appears, everything will change, and as for the second – well, he's always said it was cruel for his own parents to deprive him of brothers and sisters – so why would he wish that same fate on his own first-born?

Jill has no idea that Jack's mother would have had more children had it not been for a disorder that Jack is likely to have inherited, and will possibly be passing on to his future children. Nor does she know that his already lamentable sperm count stands to be further diminished by his tight-fitting underwear, not to mention the finish on the upholstery of his flash new car. She is unaware of the fact that the combined contraceptive pill, which she has been taking for eight years, could disrupt her cycle in such a way as to impede conception for some months after she has stopped taking it. No one has ever told her that even the most fertile woman is generally only capable of conceiving for twelve to twenty-four hours per cycle.

She doesn't even know that twenty per cent of all pregnancies (and maybe even up to sixty per cent if you include those that end too early to be confirmed) result in miscarriage – although this is nothing compared with the uncertainties she will be facing should she be so

Anatomy of a Rational Decision

fortunate as to give birth. She has no idea what this child will be like, or what kind of mother she will be, or what effect the child will have on her relationship with her husband. Of course she hopes it will all work out. She has a hunch that the odds are in their favour. When she throws away her last packet of pills that August, what she is doing is taking a calculated gamble. But when she tells her friends what she's up to, she calls it a rational decision.

She calls it a rational decision because that is what she has been trained to call it. The late twentieth century is supposed to be a time when enlightened and responsible men and women are in control of their reproductive destinies. In the old days (or so the fairy-tale goes) people had to accept the children who were foisted on them – or pay a terrible price. Nowadays, we can consider our options at leisure and make the decisions to suit our own needs and not those of society. It sounds terrific on paper, doesn't it? Maybe so, but options and choices and decisions can be hell in practice.

Why?

Well, first of all, because we don't have as much choice or control as we think we do. Science and the law may have opened many doors for the infertile and the unhappily pregnant during the past half-century, but that is not the same as saying that people automatically get what they want. Any fertility decision that involves the co-operation of public agencies will be subject to standards set by those agencies, as well as limits dictated by the law. No form of medical intervention is one hundred per cent safe.

And anyway, how many of us even know what we want? And even if we do, how can we be sure that we will go through life without ever changing our minds? In a world where fertility feelings were stable, there would be no unwanted children or regretted abortions, no requests for sterilisation reversal. In this imperfect world, most of us are in two minds not just about how many children we want, but how and when and with whom. Our plans and desires change in accordance with our changing circumstances. Even when we are convinced we're being practical, our decisions are shaped by fears, frustrations, and regrets from the past. 'Whatever I do, I'm certainly going to make sure I don't make *that* mistake again.' We are not making our decisions under clinical conditions.

Another basic fact we tend to forget when we're talking in broad terms about the importance of reproductive choice is that it takes two to make a baby. If both parties are ambivalent about their fertility, if they are too confused by their doubts and hopes to communicate them accurately, if they prefer sex to be spontaneous rather than prefaced by responsible discussion and so cannot or do not wish to apply the rules of the boardroom to the bedroom, then it is likely that any baby they happen to make together will be more wanted or more planned by one than by the other. One person's choice can be someone else's eighteen-year prison sentence. Or so it seems to the less willing partner upon first hearing about a positive pregnancy test. But these feelings, too, are fleeting. As we all know from our own experience, reluctant fathers-to-be and pregnant women who are furious at being entrapped can often turn into doting parents. How easy it is, then, for their partners to overlook their vociferous objections and go ahead to make the 'best' and most 'responsible' choice.

How can they be so sure it's the best choice? Because they have been brought up to think that rational people decide whether or not to have children in much the same way as they would decide to buy a house or a car. In fact, the language and the assumptions of consumerism could not be more inappropriate. Would you ever buy a house sight unseen? Would you buy a car without test-driving it or even finding out how much it cost? Of course not. But that, in effect, is what you're doing when you decide to have a child.

And what if you can't? If you're an easygoing, roll-with-the-punches sort of person, it's a tragedy. But if you belong to the generation that never had it so good, if you've always nurtured the illusion that reproductive choices sit patiently and alluringly packaged like so many bottles of bubble bath on a supermarket shelf, if you think of your body as a biological clock whose workings come with a twenty-five-year guarantee, then it's not just a tragedy. It's a betrayal and an outrage. 'If only we had known the facts sooner, we would never have left it all so late.' How many times have you heard childless couples blame themselves for having been lulled into a false sense of security? And yet, when it comes to knowing the facts, people like this are the norm, not the exception.

Very few of us have more than the crudest understanding of how our reproductive systems work. We may have been taught about contraception and it may seem as if we're bombarded with news about the latest breakthrough studies and scares, but this information is incomplete, inconclusive, unreliable and piecemeal. The barrage is particularly confusing if your aim is to have children rather than to prevent them.

Even assuming that we do know what we need to know, we will not be making our decisions in a temperate climate. Fertility is political. Hardly a day passes when you can open up a newspaper without finding an article about other people's fertility. If it's not abortion, it's surrogate motherhood. If it's not genetic screening, it's the world population explosion. As far as these issues may seem from our everyday experience, they affect the way we make our own decisions – and the way other people judge us. No matter when or why or how you decide to have a child – or, indeed, not to have it – your decision will be an affront to large segments of the public. If you're young, you will be seen by some to be wrecking your career chances. If you're single, you will be seen by others to be wrecking 'the family'. If you're old, you're going against nature, and if you've already given birth to your allotted 2.2 children, and you greedily desire another, you'll be instrumental in pushing the human race to the brink of extinction. When you make a 'rational' decision about children these days, you are, on account of being seen to have a choice, making a policy decision about the status of women, the future of the family, the environment, and by implication the human race.

And what if it was an irrational decision? One in three babies are unplanned, some say, while others claim it is one in two. One in five pregnancies end in abortion. Many of us are getting pregnant at times when our relationships are rocky, our overdrafts large, and our family and work commitments overwhelming. It may be faulty contraception that leads us into this predicament. It may be deliberate misuse of contraceptive devices. But it is more likely to be sporadic abandonment of contraception due to mixed feelings about having children, or the desire to test your fertility, or the need to find out how committed your partner is – or even a genuine and wholehearted longing for a child that has remained unexpressed for fear that the other party might not consent to it. The received wisdom about unplanned pregnancies is that they result from self-destructive behaviour. In fact, there are usually just as many incentives to get pregnant as there are reasons to keep it from happening.

How many times have you heard people say, 'Thank God my children arrived by themselves. I would never have got around to having them otherwise.' Have you ever heard anyone say this who does not look very sheepish? That is because he or she will have to justify not one but two puzzling decisions – the first to engage in unprotected intercourse, and the second to proceed with the pregnancy despite the arguments against it.

This is not to say you get off any more lightly if you make the other 'rational' decision – to terminate. Time and time again you'll have to defend yourself, often to hostile audiences. If you make this or any other politically sensitive choice, you may even find yourself so hard put to defend that choice, that you may end up denying any feelings that might weaken your argument, for fear of playing into the opposition's hands.

'It had to be.' 'I never even considered the other options.' 'I haven't had a single regret.' 'People told me I would feel dreadful afterwards, but I didn't. I didn't feel a thing.' These are the absolute statements you will hear from women who have had to make difficult decisions. Frequently they will go to the other extreme and castigate themselves for a 'terrible mistake'. But there is seldom a woman on the middle ground, seldom a woman confident enough to imagine in a less black-and-white way what life might have been like had she made a different decision. The imagination seems to grow blinkers after people decide which door to go through. It seems too dangerous to be hypothetical, or to entertain ambivalence after it's too late to act on it. It may be necessary to tether our thoughts. Sometimes it is too painful to dwell on the child, the life, the lovers,

Anatomy of a Rational Decision

the job, the family that might have been, and better, therefore, not to imagine ourselves pursuing a different course. Unfortunately, this often means that we are unable to imagine anyone else pursuing another course – which is another way of saying that all too often we disapprove of, discount, envy and consider ourselves a race apart from people who make decisions we would never have made ourselves.

It is our view, however, that we are all equals in front of the fertility goddess. It doesn't matter how many children we want or have or choose not to have. The urge to procreate is very strong in all of us. This is not the same as saying all people secretly desire children, because they don't. The urge to procreate and nurture can have little or nothing to do with babies. As any childless adult will tell you, there are plenty of ways of making a contribution without devoting your best years to changing nappies, and plenty of people already out of nappies who need looking after. The fact remains, though, that it almost always seems to be a blow, it almost always feels like having one foot in the grave, when you hear that, actually, you can't have children, that a choice you thought you had is no longer, perhaps never was, yours to make.

Can you even call it a choice if you didn't have 'all the facts'? Are doctors who are deliberately parsimonious with the information they pass on to patients too often making their important decisions for them? Or are they, too, making decisions without having all the facts, on account of so many patients lying to them? Are women too eager to take full responsibility for decisions they ought to be sharing with their partners and their doctors? Do men, who seldom have the last word in reproductive decision-making, have any real choice at all? These are some of the questions we'll be considering in the chapters that follow. We begin from the premise that we all fall way short of the 'ideal' when it comes to fertility. If you have ever overplanned your family, or underplanned it, or deferred a decision, or wavered, or acted compulsively; if you are haunted by visions of malfunctioning biological clocks, or if you dread the day when you have to make your final decision on parenthood, we dedicate this book to you.

We hope to convince you that you're not as bad or self-destructive or abnormal as you think you are.

But first let's take a closer look at the standards by which we judge ourselves today.

CHAPTER TWO

THE WANTED CHILD, THE PREPARED PARENT AND THE DOUBLE STANDARD

'I am sure you would not be reading this book if you were not already convinced that children should come by loving choice rather than careless chance.' So says John Guillebaud in his gently reassuring reference work on the pill.[1] Who would want childbearing in a utopia to be otherwise? Who could seriously propose the opposite, that children should arrive on earth in accordance with the laws of the roulette wheel? The ideal of the fully wanted, responsibly planned child is beyond reproach. Unhappily, it is also beyond the reach of most mere mortals. But because we are loath to air our fertility failings in public, the general view remains that the well-planned family is not an ideal, but a real possibility that any reasonably mature adult ought to be capable of managing.

The popular view, therefore, in this day of reliable contraception and legalised abortion, is that only the desperate, the ignorant, and the immature have trouble planning children. The chief domestic offenders – if you will believe what they say in the papers – are teenage mothers, who just won't listen to what their doctors, betters, and elders tell them. Much more tragic (and conveniently blurry) are the millions of poor women in the developing world who can't seem to grasp that their standard of living would soar if only they freed themselves from the yoke of perpetual motherhood.

This is not to say that their emancipated sisters in the developed world are seen to be getting it right, either. On the one hand, you have the so-called Cinderellas who retreat into motherhood because they are afraid they might fail in the real world, or because they fear the consequences of success. On the other hand, you have the Eleventh-Hour Desperadoes – the ones who were too greedy, too caught up in worldly pursuits to settle down in time. They may or may not end up in the most damning sub-category of them all – the Unsuitables. These are the women who choose to conceive even though they are single, gay, past menopause, handicapped or genetically defective.

Are they good enough to be mothers? Even the friendliest and most sensitive moral arbiters feel obliged to reassure the public on this question whenever a new scientific breakthrough brings the possibility of parenthood to a group previously denied it. The implication is that some people are not good enough to be mothers and should perhaps forfeit their right to procreate. Despite constant cries in the media about unchecked women and the disappearing nuclear family, Victorian morality rules OK whenever and wherever the law, the state, or the medical establishment have a say in the right to parenthood. A dramatic example is in the area of adoption. The drop in the number of children put up for adoption in this country following the 1967 Abortion Act has meant that the standards for adoptive parents have never been higher. Not only must they be of a certain age, of good character, in stable employment and residing in a house deemed suitable, but they must compete with an ever larger pool of equally well-endowed candidates. They must be vetted beforehand; inspected on a regular basis afterwards. Few natural parents could ever pass muster if they were judged by the same standards. Old-fashioned middle-class values assert themselves with equal force when the time comes for doctors to decide who is most deserving in infertility treatment. You often have to meet a predetermined profile, for example, if you are to qualify for in vitro fertilisation (IVF) treatment. And with very few exceptions, you also have to be in the money. We asked one woman working in family planning if she had ever considered setting up a charity for women who couldn't afford IVF. Her response was: 'Oh, they have enough children already. . . .'

This is a remark you might expect from a nineteenth-century missionary on leave from Shanghai, but from a modern day

The Wanted Child

professional? Her position is defensible, though, if you subscribe to the idea that it is irresponsible to bring into the world a child whom neither the parents nor society can afford to raise. As one IVF specialist suggested to us, anyone who cannot afford the £1,000 IVF fee can probably not afford the far more expensive prospect of a take-home baby. Although we would question connecting a particular type of bank account to the right to parenthood, many people, and especially people who have first-hand knowledge of abused and neglected children, would agree with him at least to a point. As another professional said to us, if women do now have the right to choose or forgo motherhood, if they have the wherewithal to regulate their fertility, and they're still not sensible enough to understand when they or their ilk have had 'enough children', then the time has come for society to set some limits.

And when it does, it will be bearing in mind the host of horrifying social problems that are commonly held to originate in the unplanned, unwanted, surplus child. If you believe that you can prevent crack babies or babies born HIV positive, and reduce the numbers of abandoned, abused, starving and addicted children, just by getting people to regulate their fertility better, then of course you will feel morally bound to spread the word about contraception in much the same way that your more religiously inclined ancestors might have advertised God to the heathens. But if you set up the planned child as an attainable goal, you will be leaving your disciples with the impression that any adult who conceives an unplanned, unwanted, or unaffordable child is working with something less than a sound mind.

At which point we must welcome you to the new, improved double standard. If you want to be taken seriously, if you want to command respect, then you must be seen to be restraining your procreative urges. This message has not got through to everybody, but it has a high success rate with the upwardly mobile, and with curious results. Speak to any ambitious young woman who wants to have a family 'but not yet'. After she has paid lip service to the importance of establishing oneself before attempting parenthood, she'll quickly go on to catalogue all the pleasures of life that are best enjoyed when childless. She wants to enjoy her twenties, really get to know her partner in and out, immerse herself in her job, reach a comfortable standard of living, and get travelling out of her system. All sensible reasons for using contraceptives according to the manufacturers' instructions – but for the worrying, unspoken assumptions about life post-partum.

Or should we call it the afterlife? 'When I do have children, I plan to have three one after the other – boom boom boom.' Rarely does the imagination of the tentative parent extend beyond the moment of birth. It is simply assumed that this event effects a magical transformation of character – at least in those who were sensible enough to defer parenthood until the time was 'right'. The woman who loved to linger in bed on Saturdays and Sundays will suddenly be ready and eager to give up this and all other forms of indulgence. The ruthless careerist will no longer care how many people are being promoted over her head. The exercise fanatic will be joyously philosophical about her flab, and the world traveller will adjust without effort to the tame, the domestic, and the circumscribed, carefully costed half-term holiday in Yorkshire.

Little wonder then, that the woman who was hoping to exhaust her appetite for life in time to start a family in her early thirties, decides at age thirty-two that there are a few more countries she would like to visit before she throws herself into prison, and a few more hoops she'd like to put her partner through before she throws away the key. And so the deferring begins. Although it is perfectly understandable, it is not quite rational, as it is based largely on vague but powerful fears about what parenthood will mean, working in opposition to a clear but partly erroneous image of the reproductive system as a biological clock.

'It's ticking away. But I'm sure I'll be ready when I'm thirty-five. That will give me enough time. I want two children with a space of three years between them.' Notice the speaker's confidence. She knows her powers are not limitless – all good biological clocks come to an end – but if she plays it safe and stops using contraception by thirty-five, children will appear as prearranged. If that seems naïve, it is a naïvety that has been fostered by sex educators, who promote the idea of fertility, especially fertility amongst the young, as a dangerous force that must be checked and monitored with vigilance.

Notice also that she says, '*I* will have three children.' If she counts the man out of the decision, she is, again, marching to the same drummer as most of her peers. Men might be vociferous and overbearing when discussing other people's fertility in public, and they might be the evil genies behind many institutions that discriminate against mothers, but when it comes to managing their own personal sperm pools, their record is less than spectacular. They are not commonly seen to take an interest in contraception – or to have much control over either their behaviour or its outcome. Even socio-biology has them running around sowing their seeds indiscriminately 'just in case'. Books of fertility value them for their sperm donation and their supportive role during the birth, but rarely for anything in between.

Evasion of responsibility remains a choice for men and therefore a problem. Hope remains a popular form of contraception. Even where men accept responsibility for a 'surprise' child, accepting paternity remains a challenge. The honourable man is the one who says it is the woman's privilege to choose what to do about the child, who promises to support her in her decision – and who only confides his feelings of betrayal to his closest friends once a decade in the dead of night. In public, he will work hard to keep up the front. As do we all. Because we keep our doubts and failings private, we will naturally assume, because we have so little evidence to the contrary, that few people were so foolish as to make the same mistakes as we have made.

Ask people how they planned their families, and they'll usually begin by saying they have nothing to tell. Pressed, they'll go on to say that actually they do, but that it is of little interest as it is a departure from the norm. 'I'm a special case,' they insist, but the stories – whether they result in children or not – reveal many common threads. We'll be pointing out a few of the more significant of these in the next chapters.

CHAPTER THREE

WISHES, PLANS AND EXCUSES

Why have children at all? It is no longer on to say it's a sacred duty: the population explosion has made sure of that. And it's foolhardy to assume – as people once did – that children were the best guarantee of a protected old age. In the developed world, pension plans are far more reliable than sons and daughters, who can be quick to put you into a home if you become too difficult. It is only the lucky few, with titles and business empires to pass on to posterity, who can claim to need heirs. For most of us, the decision to procreate is impractical.

Even a generation ago, men and women could say they had children because 'that is what one did' after getting married. 'We never even questioned it,' they can now say, before adding, with a gruesome attempt at empathy: 'Things are so much trickier today, aren't they? I must say, I don't envy you young people at all, with the difficult decisions you have to make!'

Certainly, it would seem like a blissful luxury to us 'young people' today to be able to go forth and multiply without having to dream up a convincing alibi. Because let's face it, they are few and far between.

This much is agreed: children, even when they are wanted, have a horrible way of slowing down careers, doubling expenses, upsetting schedules, robbing you of freedom, and playing havoc with relationships. So how to justify this strange desire? Query parents-to-be and they'll usually shrug their shoulders with a sheepish smile, and say, 'Oh, I don't know, we just wanted one.' Or, 'I've always liked children.' Pressed, they might admit – with a preface something along the lines of 'I know this sounds silly, but . . .' – that there is something deeper. They will mumble about a mysterious need to nurture, an incomprehensible desire to continue the line, a strong if embarrassing conviction that children are the highest expression of conjugal love. Time was when lofty sentiments like these commanded respect. But in the age of consumerism, such motives are suspect.

If you covet something you don't actually need, it follows that the item is a luxury. The fashionable way to describe the desire for a baby, therefore, is in terms of gratification. It may well be that many first-time parents are so blinded by family planning propaganda that they expect the wanted unborn child to transmute into a bundle of permanent joy. But that illusion quickly ends, to borrow the words of one shell-shocked new father, 'after a few days in the company of a thing the size of a hamburger that cries all the time.'

Parents looking at their younger, more foolish selves with the supercilious affection of hindsight can afford to delve deeper. 'What can I say to you?' says one woman who eventually became the mother of five. 'I just loved babies. I mean I craved them. It was an urge that dominated my life for many years.' Another woman, who cannot imagine life without her two daughters, but who misses the adored job she had to give up, not to mention the missed opportunities for travel, says: 'It has to be genetic, because there is no other way of explaining my behaviour.'

Others look back and detect hidden, and often doomed, agendas: 'I had always wanted to have children,' one man told us, 'but I was beginning to despair that it might never happen. All the women I met in my twenties and early thirties were fiercely independent and would not have dreamed of slowing down to have a child. So when I met Dot and she told me three days after we met that she wanted to settle down and have my child, I was so shocked and flattered that it never occurred to me to wonder why she was in such a hurry.'

Edith, who conceived her first child out of wedlock when she was sixteen, felt similarly desperate: 'I think I wanted to escape from a family situation that wasn't too wonderful,' she says. 'It was very much overshadowed by my alcoholic stepmother. I thought life was about getting married and having children, so there was no point in being too careful. I assumed that if anything happened, my boyfriend and I would end up setting up house, and as it happened I was right.' She went on to discover that she had walked into a trap. 'It wasn't that my husband wasn't the person I thought he was. I was not the person I thought I was. I changed, and he didn't. I did decide to have the second child. I guess I thought that was the way it was. I seemed to be following the pattern I should be following, and it wasn't until two years later that I realised I could do something about it. I wanted more than one child and it seemed like that was a natural progression. It just happened, I guess we did decide, although now I realise it was obviously totally irrational. We weren't using birth control. He didn't think it was anything wrong. Afterwards things got more difficult for me, not him.' They ended up separating when their second child was a toddler.

Does she regret having children for the wrong reasons? 'Of course not. Why would I? Give me a right reason for having a child. As far as I can see, there aren't any.' Like many other men and women we spoke to, she went on to suggest that it didn't matter what the immediate motive was, as the idea of the child before it was born had very little to do with the child you ended up with. Certainly this is borne out by the number of happy and, if anything, excessively committed mothers who reported that their desire for children began as passing fits of envy.

There seems to be no aphrodisiac more effective than the sight of a sister, or a best friend, or a colleague sitting in a hospital bed with a swaddled infant. 'I went home and cried. I was thinking, why was I the one with the career? Why was it her with a husband and me without a boyfriend in sight? Why couldn't it be me holding that baby?' is a typical explanation. So is: 'I took one look at her with the baby, and then I said to myself "Hmm, I'd like one of those for myself." '

Imagine for a moment that we are not talking about a baby but about a neighbour's sports car, a sister's new mansion, or even, God forbid, a friend's husband. Flashes of envy for such acquisitions do have a way of happening. But how long do they usually last, and how often do we act on them? If we do, can we call it a flash of envy at all, or would obsession be the operative word? And, if we set out deliberately to acquire these desirables, wouldn't we be horribly guilty from the word go about all the commandments we were breaking? The only people we spoke to who admitted to the obsessive, guilt-producing variety of envy for friends and relatives with babies were those who themselves were having trouble conceiving. Women who conceived shortly after exposure to the envy-evoking new mothers speak about the experience in a shame-free, matter-of-fact way – as if to say: 'Well, you see, there was a door in our house that was always locked, and then one day I noticed it was ajar and so, naturally, I went in to see what the room was like, and to my surprise, it looked terrific.' There is a sense of relief in their voices, a gratefulness for a motive that makes some sense, while people who cannot recall a triggering event sound troubled and inconclusive as they try to explain where their urge for children came from.

'We had a nagging sense of emptiness.' 'We knew there had to be more to life.' 'We had achieved a certain standard of living and now were ready for change.' 'We were tired of spending our Saturday afternoons buying furniture.' Anyone who remembers experiencing similar feelings will know automatically that it is a tiny little baby step from such vague feelings of dissatisfaction to an estate car packed door to door with child restraining devices. But that is not the same as explaining why this particular A leads to that particular B.

What makes people broody? This is another mystery that makes doctors shrug their shoulders helplessly. Many women describe it as an urge that descends upon them suddenly and without a cue. 'When I was sixteen,' says Eleanor, 'I had this notion wouldn't it be nice to have a child. I didn't do anything about it, as I didn't see the child as being from any particular boyfriend. And it went away. Then, in my mid-twenties, I had a boyfriend by whom I longed to have a child, but it wasn't practical.' 'It happened on my twenty-ninth birthday,' says Naomi. 'I can't explain it. It struck me like lightning.' 'I don't think I ever thought about having children when I was very young,' says Frances. 'I hated dolls, and was furious when anyone gave one to me. It was when my sisters, who are much older, had babies, and I realised actually how lovely it all is, these little personalities coming on, and it's such fun, it's fascinating, and that's when I decided.'

'I have a friend who's the same age as me,' says Karen. 'I rang her two weeks after I got pregnant and said "Guess what?" and she said, "So am I". She didn't want to have kids. I did. We were thirty-six. I think it was just a coincidence. She had just come out of a twelve-year relationship and felt very bad, and had just about sorted herself out with this new fellow who had three kids already, and then suddenly she decided she wanted a kid.'

'I was tired of playing second fiddle to my partner's ex,' says Vera. 'She seemed to be able to get away with the worst type of behaviour because he looked up to her so much as the mother of his children. They were all in mourning, the children too, and I thought if we brought a new baby into the house, everyone might start looking ahead and cheering up instead of looking back and regretting. That makes it sound like a practical decision. Of course it wasn't. It began with a desire, a very selfish desire, for something, something that I didn't have, that the ex-wife did have, and that so clearly gave her special privileges.'

'I saw it descend on my wife like a cloud,' says Simon. 'We had a perfectly happy settled life. We both had jobs we found interesting, and lots of friends and activities, and then one day I came home and she had bought a cat. The care she lavished on that cat! And the expense! The equipment! I guessed what was going to come next, and I was right.'

'I think all in all many of us have children for a selfish reason,' says Soraya, 'although we may not like to admit it. . . . I went into marriage with all the best intentions, being in love, wanting to provide a secure base for a family, and for my part I felt children were a natural expression of that love. . . . I can now admit, having been through the mill and come out the other side, that perhaps there was a deeper reason for the need for children – the need to fill the gap and heal the wounds created by my own childhood. When I first came to this country I looked back on my own childhood as very happy but gradually the mask slipped. . . .'

If these people seemed puzzled in retrospect, try talking to a few adoptive parents. They can usually remember very clearly when the thwarted desire to have children turned into an obsession. They will usually speak at length on the ways in which children have enriched their lives. What they cannot remember is *why* they wanted children in the first place.

So why *do* people decide to have children? We have established that many of the old practical reasons for families are obsolete, and also that there is no falling back on those old war-horses, Biological Destiny and Marital Duty. Any reason involving the future genetic composition of the human race must be carefully modified so as to avoid Hitlerian overtones: we don't want to give the impression that we think *our* genes are superior to anyone else's genes, do we? And then there are the doubts that feminism has cast on motherhood. Because it is now received wisdom that maternity holds women back and that many of us have children to avoid confrontation with the real world, any confession of a desire to nurture, or to turn 'love to flesh' must also be monitored, for fear of revealing Barbara Cartland tendencies. Although the language of consumer gratification is more respectable, it is known by all experienced parents to be a recipe for disastrous disillusionment if ever the desired luxury item should become a fact of life. And it's rarely one hundred per cent sincere, anyway. It's more likely to be one in a series of inadequate pretexts: 'Who knows why I arrived at the point of wanting children? It could be that I was envious of my sister. It could be that I saw a baby as a way of cementing my relationship with X. It could be that I was tired of buying furniture on Saturdays. Oh, who knows? Maybe it was just a genetic urge!'

'It wasn't my idea,' is what many people say. 'It was *her* idea', or '*his* idea'. Another common response is: 'To tell you the truth, I didn't think about it much until it happened. After that, it was simply a question of what to do about it. We never stood back and made a plan. We never envisaged what life would really be like with children.'

It becomes increasingly clear, the more modern parents you talk to, that they not only have difficulty justifying or explaining their (obviously genuine) original desire for children, but that they didn't have the faintest idea how to plan for them. Even the ones who are now happily ensconced in kitchens with Agas, the ones who seem to live to top up your tea, who never look cross when interrupted by toddlers, whose refrigerator doors are covered with animal magnets and drawings of stick figures – even these symbols of domestic success describe their early plans with the laughing derision of the war veteran for the novice soldier. 'We knew nothing, nothing, I tell you, nothing. We had some crude knowledge of a house being a necessity, and a stable relationship being a plus, but I had no experience of living, breathing children, you can laugh at me if you like, but I thought they were born sitting up. And as for the expense! It's not just the money, either. It's the time. It's the hours! It's the emotional cost! Of course I'm glad we did it, our lives would be empty without them, it wouldn't be a family, would it? But if we'd had any idea what we were letting ourselves in for . . . I don't think anyone does, really. I think deep down somewhere people realise this, and that is why they tend to ignore the facts when they're making their plans – that, or else not make plans at all, beyond saying, all right, let's fix on a number. Let's have 2.2 kids.'

Is this true of everyone? It is a fact that many of us planning families today are doing so without any recent experience of children, and that our expectations about the day-to-day routines of parenthood are unrealistic. It is likely then, that we'll have to proceed not according to plan as we move forward, but by trial and error. But does this mean that the family planning ideal never crosses people's minds? That there is no such thing as a couple sitting down and deciding to join forces and 'do it right'? Of course there is. These romantic interludes do occur. But where the promises made therein remain sacred, there is a tendency for the couple concerned to go to one of two worrying extremes. For the rigid planners, of whom more later, there will be difficulty in coping with any unforeseen event. If a miscarriage occurs, if an unnegotiated child makes an appearance after the ideal family size has been achieved, or even if a negotiated child appears at the wrong time, the response is panic, the decision made as a result often ill-considered.

And what is the other extreme? Call them the visionaries. These are the people who have a flexible but inspired idea of the kind of family they want to create. Often the vision is born out of some need for repair. There is an abusive childhood to put behind one, or a rape, or a death, or a tragic affair, or a previous failed attempt at parenthood. People starting second families are classic visionaries, their plans made both poignant and specific by their first-hand experience of domestic breakdown. But for the pure expression of the visionary credo, it is better to listen to the people who embarked on their family plan without the baggage of a bad track record.

'When did we decide to have children?' says Sarah, who married her childhood sweetheart when she was 20. 'I think it's genetic. Of course there weren't really any other options open to me – this was just on the cusp of the women's movement. But I was already that way inclined. It was a case of growing into the roles I was expected to fill. I knew I would be an excellent wife and a good mother. . . . When did I decide? Well, my husband and I had talked and talked about it from the very beginning. But the original plan was to wait for a few years so that we could get to know each other. Maybe we went through that stage faster than most. Then – I think it was about three months after we got married – we woke up one morning both knowing that the time had come. We weren't going to get any closer to each other than we already were. We saw a long future together stretched out before us. There was no point in waiting.'

The people who were able to negotiate the ups and downs of the childbearing years with the greatest ease were all visionaries something along these lines. Like Sarah, they often reported practising exemplary family planning: they discussed their feelings about children together and at length before entering into marriage. When they set up house together, they already had a schedule in place. They did not play games with contraception. Any alterations to their plans they made together. But the 'green light' decision they describe as mystical, instinctive, almost religious. 'We saw . . .' they say, 'We believed . . . we knew in our bones . . . there was no sense fighting it.' They describe starting a family as an act of faith dignified by a sense of mission. The idea of the family they'll end up with is both vivid and vague. The vision implies hardship as well as the unexpected. There is much less panic when something goes wrong – such mishaps tend to be in the scheme of things, they reason. There is also a general agreement that certain practical considerations that seem to be important to other people – like money and the freedom to travel – are not important to them. They do not talk of gratification. They talk of making a contribution, creating the type of atmosphere that will allow all family members to thrive. So what's the problem? What's to keep the rest of us from following their example? Well, for the perverse reason that they're *too* good at playing happy families. Almost all the visionaries we spoke to had five or more children.

We can't have everybody returning to *that*, can we? It takes all sorts, and it's fine if the occasional oddball couple sets out to produce a full house, but to present the large family as a model for the rest of us is to spell environmental disaster. One of the hardest tasks facing family planning agencies in the developing world is, after all, the propaganda effort to promote smaller families. We don't want to make their job even harder, do we? But before we move on with our eyes averted, it would be useful to remember that most of us in the developed world have no desire for large families. In the age of two-career marriages and consumer gratification, we are unwilling and usually unable to make the necessary sacrifices. And so we can afford to stand back and admire their vanishing virtues – if only to better understand what the smaller family is by way of contrast. Listen to what Wendy, a farmer's wife with three small children and a fourth under discussion, has to say in favour of the large family. 'They're not so intense as small families. The children aren't spoiled or left out; they're just part of the family.'

Despite her clear sense of commitment, she is quick to point out that the plan she has embarked on is more her husband's idea than hers. She felt apprehensive about starting a family, was lulled into a false sense of security on account of her first baby being easy, and said 'never again' after her second developed sleeping problems. The only reason she agreed to have a third was because they had moved to a new part of the country and her husband convinced her that a new baby would help them 'establish roots'. There were some anxieties about money, as they just manage to make ends meet, 'and I did have some population worries, but he said to me, "Some people don't have any children at all. If we bring up our children to be good people, perhaps they'll contribute to the world community in another way." We've also thought of fostering or adopting. That would be one way of helping, and it would suit us, because we like large families and so many people don't.' In other words, she has now come around to her husband's way of looking at things, but she needed persuading every step of the way.

She speaks about her ambivalence with the affection and familiarity that you might expect her to describe a childhood friend. Like bad luck and good weather, it is simply in the scheme of things, and as life unfolds you learn to get used to it. Alas, this is rarely the case for those of us who plan to have only two closely spaced children. By the time our apprenticeship is complete for one child-rearing stage, we're on to another stage for which we are entirely unprepared. We can never rest on the laurels of achievement like the mother or father of many. People who are on to their fourth or fifth or sixth child can, for example, keep a sense of perspective about the chaotic schedules of newborns. They have worked out their own way of coping. They are impervious to meddling authorities. They luxuriate in the long view: even as they rub the sleep from their eyes, they can remind themselves that there are certain advantages to this stage of development ('At least she's not putting things in her mouth yet. . . . At least she doesn't know how to roll off the bed. . . .'). They can also avail themselves of their older children, who will not just be able to help them with the care of the infant, but possibly even willing. Most of us will never know such perks. In fact, the best contraceptive of them all for most of us will be the memory of our second-born's first six months.

Those of us who limit ourselves responsibly to two children will never have a chance to move beyond the upheavals of beginning parenthood. If we're not in shock about life with toddlers who throw their food on the floor, we're in shock about life with eight-year-olds who won't make their beds, eleven-year-olds who talk back, teenagers who stay out until two in the morning. It's one surprise crisis after another. Because there is no time to develop the long view, the everyday tasks of parenthood often seem more arduous than they do to the parents of larger families – even though they will, technically speaking, have many more tasks to perform. The small family is a playground in which the intense ambivalences of early parenthood never get a chance to grow.

And there's not much we can do about it. As long as we remain committed to world population control, this will remain the modern condition. Because new parents will be coming from small families, they will have little experience of children when they start their own families. They will make laughably unrealistic plans, and learn . . . and learn . . . and learn on the job. And not just about children, either. They will also learn that men and women – even men and women who are madly in love with each other – can have disastrously different ideas about what counts for agreement, and what qualifies as a decision, when it comes to planning families.

This is what we'll be looking at in the next chapter.

CHAPTER FOUR

IMPERFECT UNDERSTANDINGS

'My son came to see me the other day for a man-to-man talk. He was upset because his wife had contrived to get herself pregnant for the second time in two years. I couldn't understand what the problem was. They had always agreed they were going to have two. I said this, and he explained that he didn't like the timing, and that really floored me. What business was this of his?'

The speaker is a man in his late fifties. His views on family planning are what we like to think of as reassuringly old-fashioned. Fertility is a woman's business: so long as she is married and able, she calls the shots. The man's job is to provide the necessary emotional and financial support.

Of course it was never that simple. But it was a popular middle-class ideal, and today, even as an ideal, it is no longer. Marriage does not imply children. It is fast becoming a woman's duty to work outside the home, rather than a privilege. She cannot expect her partner to support her should she choose to have children – and what's more, she cannot expect her partner to agree to do without *her* salary, especially since this salary may not be the supplement but the mainstay. (It is becoming increasingly common for a woman's earning power to exceed her partner's.) In the eyes of the medical establishment, and in the eyes of the law, she is still the boss. But as far as home rule is concerned, she and her partner are both likely to subscribe to the ideal of the joint decision. In other words, the man will have some influence, if not real power. At the very least he will expect to be consulted. But here an imbalance emerges.

Before we launch into generalisations, let us parade the exceptions. There are men who become broody. There are men who find pregnant women attractive, who dream of houses full of children, and who welcome the prospect of changing nappies. But in general the man will enter into family planning with a lot less interest in and tacit knowledge about babies, and a much greater interest in preserving his autonomy after childbirth, than will a woman.

'William was against the idea of children,' says Martha, 'which I probably knew before marriage. We had to go for premarital counselling because we were having a Catholic wedding. We each had to write down how many children we wanted on separate pieces of paper and then exchange them. I wrote down four and he wrote none. I ignored it. I guess I was confident I'd be able to persuade him when the time came. Then, when I turned twenty-nine, I was getting quite panicky because of all the media scares, you know, you had to start before thirty or your baby would have Down's syndrome, and so I said to William that it was time to start. And he ignored me. But after a couple of conversations, he saw it my way. My main argument with him was, look, we have a child now and I mean *now*, or else I'm leaving. Look, this is what I really want. I'm sure it was totally irrational. I didn't bother to see his side. Of course once the baby arrived his feelings about a family switched totally. It's just that he had never thought about it seriously. Most men don't.'

It may be a blanket statement, but you can't put three grown women in a room without hearing it once every five minutes. Some, like Martha, are so convinced that the man in question lacks the competence for responsible family planning that they see no point in wasting time pretending. Why humour a man into a joint decision about a subject that is alien to him? Getting him to agree to a family becomes an exercise akin to getting a toddler to hold your hand while crossing a busy street; these are situations in which it would be foolish and even dangerous to fret about etiquette.

Yes – but there *is* an etiquette of joint decision-making. Martha may not have worried too much about her husband's feelings, and she had no qualms about issuing an ultimatum, but she did seek his permission. And there is a weariness about it all – she is not taking charge for the fun of it, she is taking charge because she has no choice. She has to carry the responsibility for two people because she's the only one with the necessary qualifications. But she can't just assume, as her mother may have done, that a husband's job is to accept and provide for any children his wife might produce. She has to clear her plans with him first – or run the risk of having him run off in a huff. Here we're back in the land of child psychology, trying to make the toddler eat the food that's best for him without turning mealtime into a confrontation: it has to *look* as though the man has participated in a decision, even if this decision was nothing more than a formality.

'I always wanted to have kids,' said Jane. 'I was just waiting for a suitable donor to come along. I don't know if I would have had the balls to do it on my own. I never saw the point in having a kid for the statement's sake. I think I always envisaged some positive role for a father figure in it. God knows why I chose Sam.'

They became involved while he was breaking up with Sally, the mother of his first child, but before he had fully extricated himself. He was drinking heavily. 'We decided together that I should stop using contraception, but Sam says really that was my decision. That was just Sam being Sam. He had these fantasies when he was being adulterous that the two of us should conceive at the same time. I was a classic co-dependant at the time, but I didn't want to get sucked into his power games – Sam and his harem competing against each other, except that we weren't communicating. He has a horror of his past, and I think the only thing that is good about him is his brain.'

A point arrived when someone had to act to put a stop to things. A real baby seemed like a way to 'move on'. 'Finally, I said: "Well, how about it?" and he said "OK". I said, "I want to have a baby with you." It was rational, and he's never gone back on it.'

Meanwhile, the drama of the triangle continued. The mother of his first child kicked him out and then proceeded to get pregnant by someone else. Jane and Sam moved in together, but life was not easy. 'Things got so bad that Sam had to be committed to a psychiatric hospital, although that was a good thing because he finally got to grips with his drinking problem. This was also the year we moved to Leeds. I was commuting to London. Sam was guilt-tripping, all kinds of guilt-tripping and drinking a lot. God knows what shape his sperm was in. I still kept my GP in London. After a year of not conceiving, she made an appointment for me to go to an infertility clinic, but a fortnight before I was due to go, I found out I was pregnant. I had figured out I was getting the planning slightly wrong, and so I had made adjustments. Sam just fucked when he felt like it, and I said: "We have to do it one of these three days", and so I engineered a crucial timing, and it worked!

'It was really weird because Sam was pissed. I remember it, he doesn't. It was early December. I had just come back from London, and I remember thinking, there is nothing in the world I feel less like right now. . . .' She went ahead anyway, although it was not much fun.

Jane is not the only person we spoke to who took full responsibility with some reluctance. 'If I had waited for *him* to choose the ideal time,' says Hilda of her reluctant husband, 'we would have been in our seventies.' Says Zoe, another Helmswoman, who decided to have a child alone, 'People who don't know me think I was horribly cold-blooded about it, but really I would have preferred it if it hadn't been all me, if Neil had shown some interest in having a child. But he was just too young. He was twenty-eight at the time, and he didn't give a damn that I was thirty-eight. I remember feeling wistful that I didn't have someone else in my life, a man with a bit more oomph to him, in other words a *mensch*. But this was the choice that faced me. It was Neil or nothing. He wasn't totally against the idea of a child. He just didn't want to have to be there. He didn't want to provide support. But he was willing to go along with my plan so long as I promised he didn't have to change or pay for a single nappy.'

Problems arise when a reluctant man pairs up with a woman who is afraid or unwilling to take the initiative. 'I try and draw him into conversations about it,' says Melissa, who would like a second child before she turns forty, 'but he just won't listen. My age is simply not an issue with him. All he thinks about is his mental state and our financial standing, and neither are ever good enough for him to consider a second child as an option. What am I going to do? Sometimes I think he's just asking me to be underhanded, but if I do that, I know I'll also take the blame. And why should I, if it's something that is ultimately going to give him a lot of satisfaction?'

Some women don't seem to mind 'taking the blame'. For others, it would be unthinkable. 'I like the man to be in charge,' says Ros. 'We decided together that we wanted to move in the direction of having children, but he was the chairman of the board, if you like. He was the one who said, right, let's get on with it.' This is another common workable imbalance, and where it exists, plans tend to be sensible and logical, with practical details carefully worked out and low value given to any consideration deemed emotional. Physiological facts also count for little – this is partly due to the fact that the men making the plans have only the crudest understanding of them. But so long as the plans produce desired results, they also provide comfort and security to the Passenger Wife. However, should she wish, at any point, to suggest an alteration to the plan – because her feelings have changed, or because she has a different understanding of her situation – her Helmsman husband will often see this as a pretext to challenge his authority, and so refuse to negotiate. Where the plans are foiled by forces beyond the couple's control, he will often take the twist of fate to be proof of his own weakness – and so place himself beyond the reach of medical reassurance. Lacking the woman's understanding of the finiteness and fallibility of fertility, he is incapable of the impassive, hopeful long view. Instead he sees defeat.

This is preferable, perhaps, to what a Helmsman sees should he have the misfortune to team up with a Helmswoman. Then he sees red, and the result is war. That said, there are few perfect matches. Imbalance is the rule when it comes to planning children. Men and women tend to enter negotiations with differing levels of understanding and expertise, and firm but widely varying ideas about who should be in charge. Each couple finds its own way to share out power unfairly. Each type of working imbalance leads to a different set of problems later. But there you are. It's an unhappy fact of life that is seldom given serious consideration by family planning theorists: broodiness, like lightning, seldom strikes the same household twice in the same night. One partner feels the urgency and therefore the burden of responsibility, while the other lags behind and feels put upon and overwhelmed. This does not seem fair. Isn't it so much better when a man and a woman can grow into the idea together?

It does happen, if not as frequently as one might hope. In fact, one of the couples we spoke to that came closest to the ideal of perfect balance was a lesbian couple. Alison and Cara had both 'always known' they wanted to have children, but it wasn't until they were in a stable relationship together and 'established financially and careerwise' that they began to think about it and discuss it with friends. 'If you think about it too much, you don't do it. We just asked ourselves, are we ready? Is it a good idea? When we decided to go for it, I called about information on artificial insemination and found out what the process was, and how much it cost.' Among the many problems they had that a straight couple wouldn't have, was the decision as to which of them would try first. But they were able to decide without much trouble that this person would be Alison. 'For me, it was fear of pregnancy that was the problem, not fear of a baby. If someone had just handed me a baby, that would have been fine. That was my ambivalence.'

The planning stage for Alison and Cara was not, in other words, a straightforward exercise in strategy. It was a time during which they talked about their fears and doubts and worries and, in so doing, worked up the courage to take practical steps. Other balanced couples described a similar process. 'I had never been particularly interested in having children,' says Felicity, 'though I billed and cooed as appropriate over my two nieces when they arrived. I got married eight years ago to Owen, whose first marriage had failed, leaving in its wake two young children. We were both earning good money, and having holidays in the Caribbean, Florida, etc., as we chose, and had a "ready-made family" on alternate weekends when his children came to stay with us. An ideal situation, in many respects. However, after about three years of marriage, we both began to get a bit broody – something was missing in our life, and to our mutual surprise we discovered that we had both come to the conclusion that we wanted a child of our own. It hit us both at the same time, independently. We kept cagily asking each other, "What if . . .", and when we found that neither of us was saying "Not bloody likely", we opened up very quickly. I had up to then been very much a career woman, but I found myself disliking the pressure of work so much that I was quite willing to give it up to have a child. After talking it over at great length together, we decided that I would come off the pill the following year and see what happened.'

Colette describes a similar, and very cosy, type of gradual decision. 'When I was thirty-one,' she says, 'and my husband was thirty-six, we found ourselves both wanting change. We only imagined having children. We never envisaged what it would be like, and never decided that *this* would be the right time.' The decision evolved, she says, through long discussion. The ones she enjoyed most and found the most useful were the freewheeling talks she had with friends. In her discussions with her husband, they tried to keep on course by always returning to the same four questions: what's it about? what's important? where are we going? and what are we doing? 'Peripheral conversations are very important. It's easier if you don't have to calculate the risks, for example, what should I say because of what he might say and so on.'

But even in togetherness there are problems – especially if there is a tendency for each person to reinforce the other's inclination to defer. This can lead to the continual deferral of the decision to stop using contraception, so that negotiations go on for years longer than they needed to, and in spite of the fact that either party would have been happy for the other to give things a kick-start. Or it can lead to a continual deferral of an acknowledgement that 'contraceptive vigilance' is beginning to slip – because it is so much easier to relax standards and give nature a chance to take its course now and then, than it is to sit down and resolve all those headache-making issues that both parties agree must be addressed before they can even think of having children.

We call these deferring strategies 'chaotic family planning'. It is a popular method with women who find themselves wanting one more child than the number officially agreed upon, and amongst men and women whose career structures do not easily accommodate families, or whose many goals in life will never fit together into a harmonious whole. 'Whatever time we choose,' these people say, 'we'll be taking a heavy financial loss.' Or: 'I don't know what to do. I've put all these years into my job. And this new promotion is a one-off opportunity. But suddenly I'm wondering if I even want it. Tomorrow it might be different, but today I want a child so much more than I want that promotion. But how can I expect to support a child without that job? It's such a big decision.' The temptation, in such cases, is to arrange *not* to make it – either to drift graciously, and childlessly, from one unannounced reprieve to the next, or to invite the unholy trinity (the body, the heart, and nature) to resolve matters after the lights go out.

This brings us to our next topic: the game of contraception.

CHAPTER FIVE

WHO CONTROLS THE MEANS OF REPRODUCTION?

We'll begin with an exceptional story we hope will prove the rule. Betsy is thirty-nine, childless, broody and getting desperate. For ten years, she's been marking time in a dull secretarial job in a health clinic, waiting for her lover to leave his sexless, loveless marriage. He has promised her a child, but has said she must wait until he has left his family, which he refuses to do until both of his existing children are at university. The problem is, that takes her to age forty-two, which she fears may be too late. So she has decided to take matters into her own hands. She is only pretending that she has an IUD. But there is another problem. Her lover is a gynaecologist. He suspects a trap – or does he have proof? Did he ever conduct an investigation under the guise of lovemaking and fail to locate the thread? In any event, he has made it his business to inform himself about her cycle, and for the past four months, he has – without making an issue of it – refused to make himself available for assignations during her fertile phase. When she complains about her predicament to friends, all she gets are cries of horror. 'They say things like "Ooh, how creepy, how unsexy, it's like letting a man live under your skin!" I'm now in the invidious position of being their favourite cautionary tale,' says Betsy ruefully. 'Whenever they start to feel bad about having to take too much responsibility for contraception, they cheer themselves up by thinking about me.'

Bad or good, that is the general rule: contraception is still 'women's business'. From time to time you hear encouraging reports of men who believe that all sexually active people who don't want children to appear nine months after a given episode ought to take precautions, regardless of whether or not their partners are protected. But the more common male attitude seems to be that such tiresome matters are better left to the people who will have no choice but to bear the consequences. As Cate Haste pointed out in *Rules of Desire*, this traditional attitude was modified by the laws of necessity in the good old days when the condom was king, but it has staged a big comeback since the arrival of the pill.[1] The revival of the condom since the advent of AIDS has not, mysteriously, reversed the trend. Although only 23 per cent of women using contraceptives in this country are actually on the pill (even in the eighteen to twenty-four age groups, less than half of all women use it[2]), too many men still assume that a woman, and particularly a new acquaintance, is on the pill unless proof emerges to the contrary.

And if he discovers too late that she is not? Well, it still has nothing to do with *him*. It was her risk, her decision, not to tell him, and so her responsibility.

Even where affection for the woman is strong and the attitude not so callous, there remains the assumption that the woman, because so unequivocally in control of matters contraceptive, is clear about her intent. If she wants a baby, she'll follow one course of action. If she doesn't, she'll follow another. 'I can't keep asking her, day in and day out, if she's remembered her diaphragm,' said one man who confessed to being slightly worried about his girlfriend's contraceptive vigilance. 'If I did that she would be insulted. She would think I didn't trust her. So I've got to trust her,' he concludes. Unfortunately, if he uses the same word with her, she might interpret it as meaning that he trusts her to decide on the best reproductive future for both of them, when what he really means is that he hopes she realises that he would be shattered if she ever got pregnant.

Even those men who make love with their eyes open, and who recognise that their partners are going through 'dangerous' broody phases, will report having unprotected sex. And again, the two parties have different ways of reporting the same event. Here is Edith on her chosen method of birth control: 'David finds contraception just as unpleasant as I do, and so we practise withdrawal, with some efforts on my part to keep it from happening. If and when a child does arrive, we both accept it.'

And what does David say? 'First she talked me into two kids. Then she talked me into another two. Now she's about to try and talk me into *another* two, although just the thought of it brings on a cold sweat.' How does *he* describe their method of birth control? 'Poke and pray.'

Ask a man who has not been sterilised about his contraceptive history and you'll usually get a blank look, a shrug of the shoulders, and a curtly described strategy. 'I always use a condom.' 'I always ask.' 'I always take a condom with me, just in case.' 'I'll use a condom if I have to, but I prefer without.' This last formula, incidentally, is the most popular. Pressed about the effectiveness of his chosen strategy, a man with a few hiccups to his credit is likely to respond with another shrug of the shoulders, as if to say, well, I did my bit, didn't I? It was *her* negligence. Because he often fails to make a connection between his own sperm management and a surprise pregnancy, he will frequently see no need to alter his strategy to keep history from repeating itself.

Ask a *woman* about her contraceptive history and you'll get a torrent of information. The story will be so complex and so emotional, that a newcomer to the terminology could easily mistake the name of contraceptive devices for names of people. Although many women, and particularly young women, report having found the method that works best for them, just as many make their contraceptive history sound like a series of failed relationships. Here's Edith again: 'For a long time I used the coil. I had it removed twice to have my first and second children with David. After that it was hit or miss, method natural nothing. It was meant to be Durex, but it doesn't really happen, because I hate it. That's why it's more withdrawal, which is unsatisfactory. I hate the coil, I don't like having a foreign object inside me. The pill I just don't trust . . . all those chemicals racing round my body. I've never used the cap . . . I can't imagine that I'd ever be able to do it, and I would never get sterilised because I wouldn't want to miss the chance of another child. I guess I do play roulette now, by trying not to use the withdrawal method, but I just hope, I obviously hope David is also playing that game too, and because if he knows, it can't be such a terrible thing, can it?'

While men will complain in passing about the discomforts of condoms and occasionally the obtrusiveness of caps and (incorrectly positioned?) IUDs, women, particularly women who have had to rely on contraceptives for ten or fifteen years, favour stronger words. They hate, detest, loathe the cap, are deeply mistrustful of the pill, find the prospect of an IUD sinister, shudder at the memory of that picture of the new female condom. The first reasons offered for their negative feelings are medical. Less frequent but always strongly put when expressed is the suspicion that contraceptives are unnatural, that they curb self-expression. As one conscientious but wistful single woman put it: 'I've relied on condoms and the diaphragm, because I like to know what's going on with my body, and with the pill you don't know . . . I value myself as a physical being, and the pill suppresses the natural. I would like children, yes. I have a glowing picture of happy, secure family life. I have never trusted a man enough to be the father of my child. But there have been moments when I definitely did not want a cap in my body.'

Feelings come, and feelings go, is the moral of almost every woman's story. Each new lover, each new stage of life, presents new problems and so calls for a different contraceptive policy. Where there is a clarity of intention backed up by good communication between the man and the woman, there usually exists a strategy that can pass for rational. This is not the same as saying that it would qualify as such in court As Lorraine, a single mother, commented, 'Sometimes when a man says no he really means yes.' And what Martha says about her planning for her second child is typical of couples who want another child, 'but probably not quite yet'. She says: 'There was no conscious decision to have another. It was a half-baked effort not to have children. William, as I have explained, was now very pro children, but there was never a convenient time. Foreseeing there never would be, we thought we may as well carry on with this half-baked effort, which was, I seem to remember, some combination of rhythm and the sheath. Sounds like a dance, doesn't it? I didn't want to leave it entirely to chance, because that would probably have resulted in my getting pregnant right away. As it was, there was a gap of two years, which was fine.'

Andrea claims a similar resounding success from a 'rational' strategy no doctor in her right mind would ever condone as medically sound. 'When I was thirty-eight I had my IUD taken out, not because I wanted children, but because I knew it was now or never, and we knew that ten years down the line we would never have been able to forgive ourselves if we hadn't given ourselves the chance. But I still had grave misgivings. I was afraid that if I got pregnant I would never finish the book I had been working on for the ten *past* years. At the same time I knew in my head that it wouldn't be a baby that would stop me. It was my fear of completion that had kept me from having a family so far as well as from finishing the book. So this is what I did. I pursued the two opposite courses with equal vigour. I really do believe that I eventually got pregnant because I acted on both messages. My friends who have sat down and argued it all through and reached a firm decision haven't been able to conceive at all, and I'm sure that's why.'

What she seems to be suggesting is that the way to get pregnant is not to overcome ambivalence, but to act on it. As a theory it may be scientifically out to lunch, but it is, nonetheless, a theory that lies at the foundation of many an odd-sounding contraceptive strategy. Perhaps it could be better put. Perhaps it is that many women come to know instinctively that the prime minister of their superego is not, in the end, quite as balanced and mature as he ought to be, and therefore not equipped to act in her long-term interest. In that context, any strategy that does not follow from official policy does in fact make practical sense. Here, for example, is a woman whose first two children 'more or less arrived', but who would only want a third child 'if it came about as a result of a definite decision'. She has just taken two years off work. 'This is time off for me not to get pregnant. It's for me and my brain, not me and my body.' What kind of contraception are she and her husband using? we enquired. 'Yes, well, condoms feature on and off occasionally.'

Who's fooling whom? Most of the women we spoke to have said

they prefer not to tell the men in their lives bald-faced lies. Those women who do resort to subterfuge say they do so as a last resort, or because trust was already gone. 'Bill just couldn't accept it that there was no way I would ever have a child,' said Ruth. 'No matter how many times we went through it, I couldn't get it into his head. So in the end I gave up arguing. When no child appeared, he marched us in for fertility treatment. It was months before I was able to work up the courage to tell the doctor that I had been secretly taking the pill.'

'He was treating me like dirt,' says Tracey. 'Not only had he gone and had an affair with a woman of my acquaintance, and humiliated me publicly. But then, after he gave me a full confession and promised to give her up, he went right on seeing her. I didn't know that at the time. I thought we were both trying to work on the marriage and so I suggested another child might bring us back together. He balked at the suggestion, said the time was wrong. A few days later I saw the two of them together and figured out why. I said to myself: "Right, then, if you can do as you please, then so can I." I kept my eye on the calendar and made my plans and two months later, I am happy to say, I was pregnant with Baby Number Two.'

'He was terrified,' says Gwen. 'His reasons for wanting to postpone were all very stern and important-sounding, but they made no sense. So eventually I decided to let nature take a somewhat unusual course. When Darryl asked me, "Do you have your diaphragm in, honey?" I would say, "Yes, of course, dearest!" – without bothering to add that I had neglected to put in that all-important contraceptive jelly.'

Like most of the women we have quoted so far, she had a definite intention of becoming pregnant. But the fact remains that many, many (maybe even most) women who take risks with contraceptives do so without having planned to become pregnant. What explanations do they give?

Well, it depends on who's listening. Here are some of the standard excuses health professionals report:

> 'We were using rhythm.'
> 'The condom slipped off.'

> 'I thought I was sub-fertile.'
> 'I left my diaphragm at home.'
> 'I missed the pill.'
> 'I had just come off the pill after a media scare.'
> 'I forgot that pills and antibiotics don't mix.'
> 'I can't for the life of me remember.'

They are protestations of innocence and incompetence: either the method failed outright, or they weren't following instructions to the letter. The same stories come up when women are explaining their behaviour to friends and other non-professionals – in other words people who do not have the authority to decide whether or not they are eligible for abortion – but in this context it is not unusual to hear about ambivalence or mixed motives. Here are some typical unofficial stories:

> 'I just felt like it.'
> 'The diaphragm flew out of the window.'
> 'We were having a sort of second honeymoon.'
> 'I had a hard time remembering to take the pill because I hated the whole idea of it.'
> 'I wasn't using contraceptive jelly, because it gives me thrush.'
> 'It just seemed more natural.'
> 'That night the idea of a child seemed wonderful.'
> 'I thought if I got up to put in the diaphragm, he'd change his mind.'
> 'I thought if I asked him to put on a condom, he'd lose his erection.'

And why do men take risks with contraception? Here are some of the answers men gave us:

> 'It was her responsibility.'
> 'I just assumed she was on the pill.'
> 'I was too embarrassed to ask. I thought she would be insulted by the suggestion that I didn't trust her.'
> 'I knew it was dodgy because I was picking up some worrying signals, but I wanted to get laid, so I just went along with it.'

> 'I did ask her if she was using something, and she said yes. I knew she was lying, but because I had asked I felt I had absolved myself of responsibility for the consequences.'

And, best of all:

> 'It just never occurred to me! Because you see, a man trying to get a woman into bed has to work so hard to win her trust that it just doesn't occur to him that he might also need to trust her.'

What are the shared assumptions here? Not just that contraception is women's business, but that women hold almost all the cards when it comes to fertility. She's the one who decides when and how to contracept, whether or not to continue with unplanned pregnancies. She's the one, therefore, who must take the consequences of all her decisions. This may be as it should be, but it doesn't sit well with the ideal of family planning – the child who is wanted and planned by both parents.

So who's in charge? The woman or the man? If they're meant to share responsibility for their risks and decisions, what are the rules? Most important, how do contraceptive gamblers react to the news of a positive pregnancy test? We'll be looking at this in the next chapter.

CHAPTER SIX

HICCUPS AND SURPRISES

What is an unplanned baby? You will remember that roughly one in three babies in this country are said to be unplanned, and one in two in the US – although this slightly judgemental label is slowly being replaced by the more dignified term, 'unintended'. Although much important research has been done on unintended pregnancy, and many initiatives devised to reduce the number of unintended pregnancies, it is surprisingly difficult to get any expert to specify what criteria they use to determine unintendedness. Unintended by whom? is the first question they tend not to answer. The next is: unintended when?

How many unintended pregnancies are unwanted pregnancies? It isn't clear, because no one has seen fit to define the term. As a recent Family Planning Association article pointed out: 'The terms "unwanted" and "unplanned" are often used as if they were synonymous. However, many unplanned pregnancies become wanted just as planned and intended pregnancies may become unwanted. Also, the term "unwanted" does not convey the ambivalence felt by many women on finding themselves unexpectedly pregnant.'[1] The best working definition we have been able to come up with, and this is not from a researcher or a policy maker, but from a doctor who works in family planning, is: 'any pregnancy about which a woman expresses a regret at term or before.' By this reasoning, we would estimate that 99.9 per cent of all pregnancies we have ever heard of qualify as unwanted.

We are worried about the penchant that fertility researchers have for dichotomies. The twinned opposites 'wanted' and 'unwanted', 'intended' and 'unintended', 'planned' and 'unplanned' have an unpleasant ring to them, and bring to mind that old dividing line between legitimate and illegitimate children, the age-old and (we thought) obsolete practice of accepting some offspring and rejecting others on the basis of the circumstances of birth. Anyone who has ever been in contact with human beings of childbearing age will know that, as long as we're talking about feelings as opposed to decisions, there is no clear distinction between the wanted and the unwanted child. At one end of the spectrum is the child that is passionately desired, meticulously planned, and enthusiastically welcomed by both parents. At the other end is the unimaginable product of an unintended sexual union and an unreliable contraceptive device. In the middle are all the others and, we would say, the majority of babies: vaguely fantasised before conception, intermittently feared and regretted afterwards, half-wanted by one parent only in theory and by the other parent only in moonlight, and only sometimes negotiated.

What happens when a pregnancy occurs that is a surprise to at least one of the parents? Our experience is that no two responses are the same. How it hits a person seems to depend on how he or she feels on that particular day – about life, about the future, about the partner. Whatever it is – delight, pride, numbness, or relief; fear, panic, disbelief or anger – it will give way very quickly to another response that cancels the first one out. Some people find this emotional inconstancy so painful and confusing that after a certain point they will often say they would welcome any decision, even the 'wrong' one, as long as it brings the temperature down. 'I want to put this behind me,' they say, 'and just get on with it.'

Alas, for most of us, this is faster said than done. A lucky few can bypass hell with the help of a preformulated policy. 'I always knew, and in fact, I had made it clear to him, that I could never have an abortion', or: 'I had always said to myself that if I ever got pregnant outside a stable relationship, I would definitely have an abortion.' For us women who have no policy, or whose policies are more complicated ('I would never have an abortion unless the situation seemed hopeless, although I also think it's wrong to bring a child into the world if the father doesn't want it'), there is no reprieve. And as for men: although they have the power to make life easier or more difficult for the women who are carrying their children, they are painfully aware that they have little real say in the final decision.

The man who says, 'Oh, what terrific news! We're pregnant!' tends to be the man who has been in on the plan from the very beginning. If he never said a word about it, he is likely to have had a secret wish. There are the occasional happy cases where women – and this is particularly true if they had always had misgivings about having children and were beginning to talk themselves out of the idea – report their partners to be overjoyed by a surprise. 'When Dan and I got married,' says Eleanor, 'various people said to me, aren't you going to have a child? But I still didn't think about it. Most of my friends had school-age children by then, and seeing them didn't fill me with any desire to have children. I saw the stress. They were unable to come out, they had noisy holidays . . . not that they seemed to mind . . . but I did. It seemed to me that if you have children, these fantastic opportunities for travel just go, you lose out on the freedom to move around. You are confined . . . so I didn't want children, but I did find the problems with contraception increasingly difficult. I was taken off the pill because of high blood pressure, and then I had the diaphragm, and that became a bore, there were times I forgot it, and other times when I thought I had a rubber allergy; and after four years of marriage I suddenly found myself pregnant and rather pleased with it. And Dan was *very* happy. In a way, I think he would have liked lots of children, but he didn't get it. I didn't like the endless feeding during the night. The disruption made me very ill.'

This is what another man, Cyril, said about the unplanned conception of his now very wanted first child: 'There was a long process of not deciding. There was always a good reason for putting the whole thing off. Then my partner and I separated for a few months, which was very traumatic for both of us. After we got back together, contraception was not used. We both knew this, but it was not discussed. We were both surprised when Sandra got pregnant almost immediately. We had thought it would take us two or three years.'

Where the man is keener than the woman, he will often take a 'surprise' as a much-needed act of God. Where the man has misgivings, if not about children in general then about a child in the immediate future (and unhappily this is still more likely to be the case), the news of a surprise pregnancy can feel (in one man's description) 'like a kick in the groin'. Often he feels tricked and trapped or will suspect a plot. Says Jason, 'The first time around it was wonderful, the miracle of birth and all that, because we were happily married. But the second time it happened, I was not at all pleased. It was, I think, a mend-the-marriage baby. Of course I love my child, but I suspect his mother's motives. She was worried by then. We were not getting along, and I suspect it was all a plot on her part to keep me in tow.' Did he tell her how he felt? 'Well, I'm sure she was aware of my lack of enthusiasm. It was fairly obvious. But what was there to say?' Years later, after they were divorced, and his girlfriend ('a fantasy woman with whom I could not contemplate a normal married life') came to him with the same news, he did say something. 'I couldn't tell her what to do, but I did make it clear to her that I had no plans and never would have plans to settle down with her, and I'm sure that's why she had the abortion.' When she found out she was pregnant again a year later, he was out of the country. By the time he got back, it was too late for an abortion. 'I'm sure that if I had been here, I would have been able to kill her illusions again, and that probably would have led to another abortion.'

Although he doesn't see the resulting child very much, he is very fond of her – 'of course'. The idea that he might have been able to talk her mother out of having her has no effect on his paternal feelings. 'With my ex-wife, it would have been different, because ending a life would have meant a lot to her. With my girlfriend, I don't think there is the same significance. She comes from a wealthy family that doesn't respect life much. You keep some people, you throw others away. That's how it works with them.' As far as he is concerned, the fact that the child is genetically half his is irrelevant. It is her body, her child, her abortion. Like many men, his concern when confronted with a surprise conception is not the baby but his understanding with the mother. If he's already inside a marriage, then there's not much he can do beyond staging an overtime ban. ('I'll do my best to cope, but don't expect me to do anything extra or show any enthusiasm.') But if the relationship is still undefined, and if he senses the woman has plans, he'll consider it his first duty to disabuse her of illusions. He will be careful to let her know exactly what kind of support she can or cannot expect from him.

Looking at this type of situation from the woman's side, the man's policy statement will often be the first hard news she has ever had about how serious he is. If the news is bad, it will now be the woman who feels tricked and trapped. Imagine, for example, a woman who has allowed herself to be seduced by an older, married man who has told her how desperately unhappy he is, and how he longs for a new life with her, if only he can find the courage to be selfish and put his own needs before his children's. For six months, they have been building elaborate castles in Spain while having lunch-hour sex, sometimes with precautions, and sometimes (they are both aware) without. Perhaps he has even said to her that he wishes something would happen to 'force the issue'. Perhaps she has been naïve enough to take him seriously. How will she feel if he reacts to the news that she is pregnant by telling her that whatever she decides, she had better be clear that their affair is getting out of hand and must come to a close? Even if she had always wanted a child, even if she has no qualms about having a child on her own, she will feel that she has been left, literally, holding the baby.

But people who are discussing the fate of a surprise baby tend to talk only in the vaguest terms about that baby's possible future. It rarely goes beyond, 'How will we cope? Who will take care of it? Where will we find the money?' The real concern is what is going on in the here and now – what the pecking order happens to be in the given household, what the understanding is between the putative mother and father (and, if they are underage, what the understanding is between them and *their* parents) – and how they and their supporting cast believe the status quo will be challenged by the baby's arrival. To quote Frances, who went through agonies as the result of an inopportune pregnancy, 'It's hard to say what I would decide if I had it all to do again, because he's here and he's a person now, and I think that's the point, that's what you have to remember, you're talking about other people, and that's the first thing you notice when they're born, this entity arrives, and you think, who am I to . . . I knew the minute he arrived, bang, I knew that person. I knew I'd recognise him anywhere and that was it, that was the core of it. . . .'

But as she herself would be the first to point out, that is only the core of it after the moment of birth. So long as the baby is an unknown quantity – and this is true even for women who talk of babies being alive from the moment of conception, and who have seen the fetal heart beating on the ultrasound screen – the baby remains a symbol. To the unconsulted, unaccepting father (or, in the case of a teenage pregnancy, the shocked grandparent) it can be a big blob threatening all hopes for future domestic harmony. To the unthanked mother, it can be a naked light bulb that exposes every corner of her shamefully irresponsible fantasy life for all to see, and that makes the future look grimmer than she ever thought possible. Even if she half-wanted this child when it was hypothetical, even if she half-planned it, a surprise pregnancy will cause her to examine her motives, her ambivalence, and her future plans in a cruelly harsh light. To quote Frances again: 'Having two children and being at uni was very difficult, and I kept thinking, are we going to have another child, or aren't we? We reached a point – my second must have been eight or so – when I thought, we're obviously not because life isn't working out that way, and I really want to go back to work now, and so I went and took careers analysis, I went up to London and took a whole day and spent a lot of money, and ten days later I found out I was pregnant. I had actually started giving away all the baby stuff. I had held onto it for a long time, and then when I reached that point of saying, actually, we're not going to, I became pregnant. I must have been pregnant when I went up to London, so yes, the baby was an accident, but if he had been three months earlier, he wouldn't have been an accident, he would have been a half-hearted attempt. It was very traumatic. I couldn't decide what to do. I agonised, and then, just after we knew, my husband had a big bust-up with his

Hiccups and Surprises

partners at work so it was very traumatic, the whole thing, but it all worked out. It's quite extraordinary.

'I don't think I could have had an abortion, personally, because of my Catholic upbringing, which is much stronger than I would like to think,' she continues. 'I would never dream of saying to anyone else that they should or shouldn't, but myself I think I would feel pretty terrible about it. I did consider it that time because I was so sort of shocked by the whole thing, because I had mentally got myself back to the idea that I was going to work and to get myself trained, so I was sort of stunned by it, and I suppose till I'd seen the doctor about my specific medical worries I had an open mind about it, but I decided not to do it. I did have another scare, when this third child was two. I must have skipped an egg or something, and that time I was very scared and would have considered an abortion then, I think, because I don't think we could have afforded another baby then.'

Many other women from Catholic backgrounds, and even some women who were still practising Catholics, made similar comments about abortion. They didn't think they could have abortions, but they had had occasion to seriously consider having one. In other words, people who are grappling with the prospect of an unintended pregnancy often use the *idea* of abortion as a let-out clause – even if they would be extremely reluctant to actually have an abortion. The availability of abortion allows them to free themselves – at least theoretically – from biological destiny. It allows them to choose a child out of their own free will, rather than be forced to accept it against their will. Thus, through the magical intervention of misleading rhetoric, the unplanned, unwanted child transforms into a planned and wanted one.

The same thing happens when a woman wants and fears a child in equal measure, or shies away from the prospect of 'playing God'. Here again the *availability* of choice allows her to make some kind of pact with herself, and also limits the scope of her decision, thereby absolving her of the sin of hubris. Listen to the story of Kitty, who was thirty-eight and single when she became accidentally pregnant for the third time. She had terminated the other two pregnancies, in both cases because she was not in a stable relationship, and because she was convinced that a child would wreck her life. On this occasion, however, she felt differently, not because of any feelings for the father, whom she had met while on holiday in the Far East, and whose name she had forgotten, but because she had lost both her parents very suddenly two years earlier. She had a longing for family, but she had little confidence in herself as a parent, and she also feared for her elder sister, who had been trying without success to conceive a child for years. She didn't know what to do, so she summoned an old friend for the weekend and put the question to her. This friend said she could not tell Kitty what to do, but she assured her that she would be a good mother. It happened to be the Saturday of the Grand National, and it also happened that a 100-1 outsider was running that was named after the place where the baby had been conceived. Kitty put fifty pounds on the horse and said that if it won, she would go ahead and have the baby. The horse won, confounding all predictions. The friend was badly shaken. Imagine her surprise, then, when she mentioned the Grand National in passing to Kitty a few months after the child was born. 'Which Grand National are you talking about?' Kitty asked. It emerged that she had forgotten the circumstances of her decision. As the details returned to her, and she conceded that it had indeed happened, Kitty's words were, 'Oh well, then, it was meant to be.'

When choices seem too big, the only way to proceed seems to be to trick yourself into believing that it wasn't your choice to make in the first place. It doesn't matter if it's all a game, if it succeeds in its main objective, which is to quell the terrible fears that a pregnancy can cause in a woman if she lacks the protection of a preconceived plan. Men don't usually have to worry about the final choice landing on their doorstep, but the same primitive fears about pregnancy seem to affect them, too. One of the ways they cope with these fears when they occur is to disconnect. Whatever the strategy, it is unlikely to sound logical to the bemused bystander or the unamused mother of the child, but again, perhaps the only important thing is whether or not the strategy quells the panic about the prospect of being a father.

Consider this story about Antony, whose girlfriend told him she had conceived his child during the last month she cohabited with her

Hiccups and Surprises

husband. She had had sex with her husband too during that cycle and, although the dates would indicate that *he* was the father, and not Antony, she knew 'in her bones' that Antony was the father. Antony was not convinced but generously offered to support the child even though the other man was most probably the father. When the child, a carbon copy of Antony, was born, he still persisted in thinking of him as the other man's child. This did not keep him from providing all the support he had promised, and more. Nevertheless, when the child was about six months old, Antony's girlfriend decided to have the infant genetically tested. The results confirmed that Antony was the father. Delighted, she left a message to that effect on his answering machine. When Antony came home and heard the message, he keeled over and fainted.

Fatherhood had been a cinch for him. It was the *idea* of paternity that caused him distress. He could stay on track for as long as he could fool himself that the child had nothing genetically to do with him. Or was the problem in Antony's case the realisation that his happy, harmless little game of denial was no defence against the ever growing, ever more intrusive arm of science?

Up until now we have been looking at how people imagine, plan and conceive their children in the privacy of their own homes and bedrooms, and even inside their heads. Whatever training they have received about contraception, they have been able to use or misuse it without censorious supervision. Feelings come and feelings go, fantasies form and reform, stories are constantly being revised and rewritten, and even if surprise pregnancy does occur, the first concern is rarely the unknown quantity that is the source of the panic, but the ways in which it is imagined that the unknown quantity will change the lives of its parents.

The rules of engagement change from the moment those parents walk into a doctor's surgery. It doesn't matter if they are there to ask for an abortion or to book in for antenatal care. From this moment on, they are part of the public record. There will always be official witnesses. There will also be an expert opinion, a standard of conduct, a set of procedures, and a framework that keeps feelings in perspective, makes fantasies look silly, and accepts only those stories that are consistent and plausible. From here on in, the parent-to-be will be living a double life. The public life will, ideally, be following the dictates of good medical practice and will oversee all serious decision-making. The private life will continue to operate according to its usual emotional logic, with the difference that every event, every game, every negotiation is further complicated by the forays into the world of medicine. If it weren't for the advances of science, we wouldn't have much choice when it came to reproduction. But it is the clash between the scientific method and the logic we have traditionally used in such matters, that makes our medical decisions so difficult, and produces such odd after-effects.

CHAPTER SEVEN

WHOSE DECISION IS IT ANYWAY?

First let's stand back and survey the menu of services on offer. If we don't want to get pregnant, there is contraceptive advice and provision. If we can't get pregnant naturally, there is fertility treatment. When we have managed to conceive, there is antenatal care, genetic testing for the high risk mother, and ever improving technology for the management of miscarriages, premature births, and problem deliveries. If we decide not to go ahead with a pregnancy, there is therapeutic abortion. If we decide we don't want any, or any more children, there is sterilisation. And if we find any decision facing us particularly daunting, there is counselling. Who could ask for more?

Anyone who reads the papers knows that there is plenty of room for improvement. Even where there is no hint of malpractice, there are many complaints about procedures that fail to accommodate patients' needs, professionals who treat the body rather than the person, who fail to monitor their prejudices, who do not give the patient enough time or enough information to make considered decisions. If the medical service became more patient-centred and accountable, the argument goes, these problems would disappear.

And so they would and should. However, there are other problems that such streamlining of services would not solve and could even exacerbate, and these come from an almost universal misunderstanding as to how normal people feel about fertility, and how these feelings affect the way they go about making their fertility decisions. What doctors and reformers share is an unexamined faith in the idea and desirability of choice. To question it would be to undermine the philosophical foundations for both camps. What we would like to suggest is that *not* to question it is to grow blinkers, and therefore to perpetuate a menu designed for a patient who does not exist.

Let's begin with the most controversial service of them all: abortion. It is there, from the doctor's point of view, in order to protect the woman's physical and mental health, to spare her the tragedy, and society the cost, of a genetically defective child, and (for some doctors, anyway) to remedy contraceptive failure. It exists, from the feminist's point of view, as the guarantee of autonomy. Throughout history, women have been kept in their place because others controlled their fertility: it therefore follows that we must take control of our own fertility if we are to be free. In this scenario, doctors are necessary but suspect allies in the struggle against the pro-life movement, which insists that the rights of the unborn are more important than the rights and needs and problems of the mother.

The lines of the battle determine the terms of debate. When we argue about abortion, we focus on safety and morality and rights, the standards of care and the likelihood of physical or emotional aftereffects. We have so much invested in our ideological position (whatever that happens to be) that when we hear a case history that doesn't fit into it neatly, we are often too afraid to take it in. To consider the implications of that history would, after all, be to play into the hands of the enemy. Maybe so, but it also means that we fail to observe what is going on underneath our noses.

Let's remind ourselves of the statistical bare bones. One in five pregnancies in this country ends in abortion. One in three women of childbearing age has had a pregnancy terminated. What did these women have to go through? How did they arrive at their decisions? What kind of support did they get? How did they describe their ordeal afterwards? If it was a traumatic experience, why? And what do the experiences have in common?

There is no consistency as far as personal verdicts are concerned. Some women are insistent that the process was straightforward, unemotional, and easy to forget about afterwards. Others talk of long depressions afterwards and deep regrets. Women who have had one abortion when very young and then another after their family was 'complete' say there was a difference between the two experiences. In the first instance, they knew little of pregnancy, life, and often even the father, and so there was no problem. In the second, they not only knew and loved the father, but knew what his children looked like, and so the decision was a much greater struggle and much harder to recover from. This would seem to suggest that abortion is easier to endure in early life than it is later on, but no rules hold fast when we focus on emotional responses: there are plenty of young women who grieve for years about an abortion, especially if they come to the conclusion that they did it not for themselves but to appease somebody else.

So if it is impossible to predict who will look back on an abortion as a right or wrong decision, what do these women's accounts have in common? There is, first of all, a vehemence with which they describe the dilemma they were faced with. 'I had no choice', some say, usually meaning that the penalties of having a child were so high as to be unimaginable, while others say: 'It was me or the baby and I chose me', usually meaning that the abortion was for them a desperate act of self-preservation. The second thing that is common to almost all accounts is the deep and protective empathy these women have for any other woman who has been faced with the same decision and an anger at the insensitivity of pro-life campaigners. 'As if they have any idea what a woman goes through before she makes her decision!'

And here is the key. What *does* she go through? To what degree is her ordeal private and to what degree a committee effort?

Meet Nancy and Bob. They have known each other for two years. They have discussed the possibility of having children together, but he has told her he is not ready for a decision yet. He isn't sure their relationship is stable enough for the long haul. He doesn't know his own feelings. It's not that he has any real interest in seeing other women – it's that he wants the right to see other women, in theory, if not in practice. He doesn't want to make any promises he won't be able to keep. 'That's fine for him to say!' thinks Nancy to herself. He's happy to take all the support she can give him, but what is he willing to give her in return? Sometimes it seems as if things will go on like this in limbo until she does something to take charge. She has been using the diaphragm. Suddenly it begins to look like a device other people have talked her into using for their convenience and her oppression. On her safe days, she stops using it and finds sex more exciting than ever. She notices he takes no notice of its presence or absence. It seems to her that he might be silently asking for her to solve all his problems by getting pregnant. She stops using her diaphragm altogether. The knowledge that she might possibly be pregnant makes her feel secretly special, and so better equipped to cope with the little everyday degradations of her situation. All this changes when it starts to look as if she might actually have pulled it off.

For two weeks, she can't even think about it. Buying the test is one of the hardest things she has ever done. When it turns out to be positive, her first words to herself are: 'Well, you've really done it now.' It is another two weeks before she rings up Bob and tells him that they must meet urgently, as she has something very important to tell him. The only reason she takes this step is because she tired of thinking up other explanations for her lethargy, her nausea, and her sudden aversion to coffee and alcohol.

What should she do? She is terrified by the idea of a baby but even more terrified at the prospect of an abortion. How will Bob react to the news? How will she explain her behaviour? If honesty is the best policy, she should explain the various resentments that led to her stopping contraception, but what if he says that she misunderstood, that he was not making a silent plea for her to become pregnant because he was tired of making decisions? If she is going to be honest, she will have to also tell him how very different her feelings are now that she actually is pregnant. But if she does, she will be giving him the ammunition he needs to talk her into an abortion. If what she wants is to talk him round, it may be better not to blurt all that out, but to manoeuvre things in such a way that he, too, decides he wants this baby. In which case, she had better make sure she knows that she does too. Or is she after a commitment from him? Is this poor unborn baby nothing more than a pawn? How will she feel if he is unwilling to make a commitment to her even though she is pregnant? Will she still want the baby if she knows she may be bringing it up alone? First things first, she decides. She needs information before she tackles that one. When she tells Bob the news, the first thing she says is that his feelings count too, and that she will have an abortion if he doesn't want the baby.

But this approach doesn't work. Bob can't even begin to think about the baby itself. He is too suspicious that she is trying to manipulate him. Why should he have to decide about a baby he never wanted to have in the first place? he protests. He can't force anyone to have an abortion. He doesn't believe it's right to tell a woman what to do with her body. His greatest concern, therefore, is limiting the commitment that this deviously engineered pregnancy is luring him into. He says okay, go ahead with it so long as you realise that I promise you nothing. Even with this large exit clause, he feels entrapped. And Nancy, too – she feels that she has been manoeuvred into a position where she has to accept all the responsibility and all the blame. So she tells him if that is his attitude, she's going to have an abortion. 'And I hope you realise that half the couples who have abortions split up within the year,' she sobs. He shrugs his shoulders. 'The least you could have done,' she says, 'is hold my hand while I go through with this.' She half hopes he will break before the day of the abortion arrives, and stop her at the door, and say that he can't let her do this to their child. But what if this doesn't happen?

By the time she makes an appointment with her doctor, she will be eight weeks pregnant. By the time she sees the doctor, it will be closer to nine. If she requests an abortion, and her doctor consents on condition that she agrees to an hour of counselling, followed by a second consultation with him the following week, she will be ten weeks pregnant by the time she is referred to the hospital. This means that she will have had what is considered to be ample time to consider her decision carefully. Her period of indecision (and pointless morning-sickness) will have been mercifully short, and the chances of emotional and physical trauma lower than they would be otherwise, as first-trimester abortions are usually quick and safe and do not always require a general anaesthetic. But think again. This timetable allows her two weeks in which to make what could be one of the most significant decisions of her life. How will she be spending these two weeks? Feeling and hiding nausea, castigating herself for 'getting into this mess', wanting the baby, hating the baby, fearing the consequences of an abortion, fearing the consequences of a pregnancy outside wedlock, wondering why Bob is acting like a zombie and pretending the problem has nothing to do with him, wondering if they'll split up if she has an abortion, wondering if he'll leave her in the lurch if she doesn't, asking herself if it even matters if this is what he's like in a crisis, pretending to the world at large that everything is absolutely normal, and then, behind closed doors, thrashing things out with her cast of chosen confidantes. During the first week of deliberations, this will consist of Bob, and, because his response has so upset her, three women she knows who have had abortions, two of whom think Bob is no good. Her mother will also involve herself, having dropped in one afternoon, found her crying, and guessed. What we have now is a private melodrama, six over-emotional characters in search of a resolution. Each one has a different set of vested interests, a different position on abortion, and a different standard of behaviour. How they behave will determine what she tells her doctor she has decided she wants. If they scare her by isolating her emotionally, she is likely to panic and have an abortion to win them back. If she interprets the same ploy as an attempt at coercion, she is likely to decide not to have an abortion just to spite them. It's impossible to predict.

In this case, let's imagine that she does decide she has to have an abortion. She's still in full-time education: a baby now would ruin her life. If it's a choice between her life and a baby's life, she's choosing her life. As far as she's concerned, Bob is history: she is furious at the way he has been acting over this past week. She is not up to the prospect of being a single mother, especially since she's never going to speak to her own mother again. At the same time, she is terrified at the prospect of an abortion. What if she regrets it

Whose Decision is it Anyway?

afterwards? She knows she can't go through with it if she thinks about the baby too much, and so what's the point of sharing her feelings with the doctor? She's thought about it. She knows what she has to do. Now she has to find the courage to do it. But the doctor insists on an hour of counselling, and the counsellor believes that the women who come through the experience of abortion with the least emotional scarring are the ones who are fully in touch with their grief before they proceed.

How will Nancy react to the counsellor's attempts to break through her already shaky defences? Will these attempts be subtle? clumsy? value-free? laden with prejudice? What choice will the counsellor secretly want her to make? Will Nancy guess the bias? Will she find this bias a relief, and an invitation to let someone else play God for her, or will she be angry about the attempt at intrusion and react against it? It's impossible to tell. Tune in next week. What we have, in other words, is act two of the same drama.

We are always discussing abortion as a private, intensely personal choice, a responsibility too weighty to share, a painful decision we must make of our own free will. But in fact the decision can be very public. Most women find themselves making it on a stage. Because, like all powerful drama, it involves the protagonists stripping themselves of pretensions, revealing their characters, betraying trust, and complicating the action with their hidden agendas, it is a draining experience. Because it involves authority figures and health officials, it is also shaming. 'You're never the same again after you've had a termination,' one drama-scarred and keenly empathetic abortion counsellor told us. 'You might recover outside but inside you're never the person you were before.' Why might that be, we wonder? How much of the trauma is due to the fact of the abortion? How much is due to the nightmare rituals that surround the decision-making? And how much is due to the fact that the woman subsequently takes full personal responsibility for what could be seen as a community decision? After all, when a woman decides not to have a baby, it is often because her circumstances will not accommodate a baby. If schools and employers were more flexible, if families were less panicked, and partners were more forthcoming with support, her decision might have been different. So why does she say 'I' had an abortion instead of 'we'? Or more to the point, since we do not want to suggest that the decision should be taken away from her, why does she say she had to choose between her life and the baby's, instead of saying that she made the decision she did because she got such a negative reaction from her nearest and dearest that she didn't have the heart to foist an unwanted baby on them?

Speak to a woman about her abortion and sooner or later you'll begin to feel as if you're sharing the room with a large, hostile audience. The woman acts as if she's speaking from the isolation of a spotlight. It doesn't matter if she says '*je regrette tout*' or '*je ne regrette rien*'. Her tone is almost always defensive. Even if she has catalogued the experience as 'just one of those things', the eyes in her immobile face will look worried. Even if she did not suffer as the result of an abortion, she has learned that there are plenty of people out there who think she ought to have suffered. 'They even had the nerve to tell me how I was going to feel afterwards. As if *they* knew.' 'I have never felt so exposed, so alone.' These are the words of women who feel they have been singled out for public humiliation. And this despite the fact that only a very few people in their social circles will ever even know that an abortion took place.

What we're talking about here is shame, with all its attendant cover-ups. The general public must not know what happened to our heroine. This is for her own protection, because for many she is today's scarlet woman – except that her sin is not adultery, but abortion.

People who have been disgraced feel obliged to give an accounting for themselves. Their stories give shape and meaning to the crisis they went through and so imply either that the rational has prevailed, or that whatever decision they took was somehow meant to be. Here, for example, is a moving and clearly honest account of a difficult abortion published anonymously in a newspaper:

> '. . . Justifications alone were not enough to carry me
> through the experiences unscathed. They were not enough to
> shield me from the intense regret and grief which grew over
> the years. They were enough to carry me through the offices

of a pregnancy advisory service, where I sat in a waiting room with a bunch of girls and women each clutching their own justifications. They were enough to carry me through the medical examination, where a woman doctor explained that a tube would be inserted in my womb and the "products of conception" vacuumed out. But they were not enough to carry me through the moment I awoke after the operation. My waking thought was not that "the products of conception" had been swept from my womb. It was "Dear God, my baby is in an incinerator." I had committed the most unnatural act a woman could commit: I had killed my child. I have never totally forgiven myself. . . . In the end, despite the raving and obscene pamphlets issued by pro-lifers, despite their pictures of an eighteen-week-old fetus sucking its thumb in a womb and a mangled mess of fetal limbs after an abortion, I have not changed my politics, nor my belief that I had a right to do what I did. In the end it was *my* body, *my* baby, *my* abortion, and *my* right to choose. Putting myself back in my twenty-one-year-old shoes I can still see that the choice I took was the only viable one open to me. Of course, so much of what I have said is confused and contradictory. But then abortion is a confused and contradictory issue – ask any woman who has had one. But if I am going to be honest then I must say that no single act in my entire life has ever made me feel the guilt the abortion made me feel.'[1]

There is an air of tragic inevitability about this decision. And it convinces.

But where people are able to remember the minutiae of the decision-making process, they paint a very different picture.

Take Heather, who was thirty-five years old when she was hit with a pregnancy scare. She had two school-age sons and a very demanding full-time job without which it would have been impossible to pay the mortgage. She had always been very careful about contraception – in fact, she had only had unprotected sex three times in her entire life. Two of these occasions resulted in her (jointly planned) children, the other was after she was raped at the age of nineteen. It seemed like the obvious choice to have an abortion in that instance, but she still found the experience traumatic. 'It sounds so stupid . . . you've been raped, you don't want the baby, you want to end the pregnancy, and yet as soon as you have ended the pregnancy you just want the baby. . . . It's total insanity, there's no logic behind it, except that it's the natural mother's urge to protect the unborn child. . . . I did feel it was the right decision but also a wrong decision. There was no right decision to make, but I made it, lived with it, it was the lesser of two evils, and I suppose I wanted that child replaced in a ridiculous way. I understand the logic behind it myself. It was James who basically said, no, don't replace that child, we're going to have the right child, our child in the right time, and that was it, and eventually I felt that actually that was a much better way. . . . We would have our children, not the replacements for an appalling tragedy that happened when I was nineteen.'

And so they did. She knew, when she brought her second son home from hospital, that she and James had accomplished what they had set out to do, and that their family was now 'complete'. But the tragedy of the rape and the abortion came back to haunt her when she had her pregnancy scare. 'I lost my coil and my period was late. *What* a combination. The doctor said, "Well, how do you feel?" and I said, "I can't make a right decision, I can't have a termination, and I can't have a baby. If I had the baby, I'd have to take my dyslexic son out of his special school, and I can't cope with destroying his ability to achieve. I can't make that decision, and I can't have a termination, don't ask me the question because I don't have the answer." And she said, "We'll get an early pregnancy test done, but at this moment, I'm concerned about your personal life. You have a coil that's gone walkabout and could turn up anywhere." '

As it turned out, they managed to find it, and the pregnancy test proved negative. But because the scare lasted only four days, Heather has a very clear memory of the emotional turmoil it caused. She thinks that may have been the point at which she well and truly accepted that she could never have another child. 'It was probably an economic decision, because of my dyslexic son's educational needs, but the decision at that point was "Don't ever make me have to make that decision again." It was a "logic" no. Emotionally I'm not quite sure because I don't allow myself to think about it. James' view was simple and logical. There had to be an abortion. "We cannot have this baby," he said. He is a very logical person, non-emotive driven. He makes all his decisions with his head. And I adjust to live with that. He has a very analytical approach to life whereas I have a very emotive approach to life. That's probably why we make such good decisions as a pair. I was angry. I understood that what he said was absolutely right, and it did make me focus on the fact that I couldn't have the baby, but I resented it – and knew he was right. Big decisions are always like that – muddled and confused. I was frightened I was going to have to make the decision. It was fear of the decision!

'Once I had made the decision I probably would have just got on with it, but to make the decision, it put me through hell for three days. It was only three days, but it was a lifetime. If the scare had continued, I think he would have pushed through the logical argument, because at the end of the day he was logically right. It would have been my choice. I think in the end I would have followed his logic. Reluctantly realising he was right. I know all the hell I went through that he will never understand, and I don't know if I would have been able to persuade him emotionally about how I felt about it so that he . . . I just know I never want to have to make that decision. . . . In the end he would have decided, but I wouldn't have let him make it with me. . . . I knew where he was coming from and logically he was right, but he didn't have to live with the emotional angle. In the end I would have tried to do it totally on my own without influence and then tried to persuade James to support me. I'd like to think he would have gone along with my decision, although in reality I don't think he would have, unless I had followed the logic route.'

If she had had to have an abortion, she says, the decision would have been much harder than when she was nineteen. 'That decision was easy, logically. This one would have been different because there was a family unit. All sorts of tragedies and calamities appear in your life and you do find a way round it. People do lose their jobs and do change and you readjust and carry on. . . . I never teased myself with the thought that it might be a little girl. It was just the agony of, "God, I'm going to have to make another decision." '

Because she sees herself as all emotion, and her husband as protecting her from herself by being all head, she sees the ideal joint decision as the perfect balance of the rational and the emotional. If her account is full of contradictions it is because they never did have to make the decision: the crisis ended before it had to be resolved. It is clear from her account that she would have had great difficulty carrying through any course of action without his seal of rational approval. Even though she says over and over that there were things he was not taking into account – the agony she went through after the first abortion, and the possibility that the trauma she might suffer after a second abortion could be even worse – she remains desperate for him to remain in charge of all family decisions. What she fears most is having to do again what circumstances forced her to do when she was nineteen – having to take sole responsibility for a decision, and shoulder all the guilt. All the women we spoke to who had been faced with crisis pregnancies spoke of this fear of loneliness, this dread of having to take sole responsibility for a life-or-death decision. While they talk of the importance of joint decisions, what they often seem to need is unconditional support. The honourable partner is still the one who says, 'Whatever your decision, darling, I'll be there next to you, holding your hand.'

This was more or less what Donna's husband said when she became accidentally pregnant. 'It was quite shocking. I was over forty. We were using condoms. I assumed I would be safe. We had been discussing the possibility of sterilisation, but without pressing urgency. There seemed to be no need.' The pregnancy came just after Donna had gone back to work, partly because of financial difficulties, partly to get back into the swing of things in the real world. Their three children were all in full-time schooling. 'The family was complete.'

'I had had an abortion before I got married after an early brief encounter. There was no question about it. And it was easy, like having your tonsils removed. It's easy when the other half of the baby is someone you don't know. This time, though, it was agony. There was no good reason to have another baby, but I also knew that this baby probably wasn't so different from my three boys. I spoke to a number of close friends about it. Some were sympathetic, some were shocked and some were on the fence. My sister suggested I wait a long time to be absolutely certain. She didn't want me to make a snap decision. She told me I was always happiest with a little baby around. But I also knew babies turn into horrible children, and that I had made mistakes with my eldest because I didn't have enough time for him. I knew if I had another baby, all aspects of family life were going to suffer. I had a gut feeling about it. My feeling was no, not to wait like my sister advised, but to make a decision soon and get on with it. I didn't want the pregnancy advancing. Already by eight or nine weeks, there were too many familiar feelings. I wasn't going to waver, with a life growing inside me, while I said, "I wonder if I'll have it or not?" That didn't seem right. Nick said he was slightly more than fifty per cent in favour of having the baby, but the decision was mine. If he had been more assertive, if he had exerted any pressure either way, it would have been the road to a nervous breakdown. Although I don't know – if he had come in and said, absolutely not, that would have been interesting, because I'm contrary. I would have been angry and maybe had it to spite him. And if I had had a partner who really, really wanted the baby and I went ahead and had it, I might have hated him or hated the baby. It's a risk. But as it turned out, I had lots of support and so it went smoothly. We kept it quiet. I can't read the abortion press. I have no interest in the pro-life case, in fact I find it quite sickening. They just don't know what they're talking about, and I do, I know all sides. I can't listen to people who haven't this experience. There was a prolife campaigner outside the nursing home where I had the abortion. A bloke on his own. He hadn't a clue what agony I'd been through. As if I had said, let's nip up here for an abortion. The assumption is that a woman has no feelings for the baby. But that's not the case. I came to my decision after a great deal of soul-searching. At any other time, I would have been vocal with this pro-lifer, but in the circumstances, I collapsed into tears. It's nobody's business but the woman's. Although the partner can be consulted, the decision should be hers. Even though he is an equal parent, he doesn't have equal say, because it's her body. When other people interfere, it's yet another case of, "Oh, women can't work these things out for themselves." '

But what kind of unconditional support is the right kind of unconditional support? Another woman we spoke to, a doctor's wife who became accidentally pregnant under similar circumstances, told the following story with some resentment: 'I gave him the news at a restaurant and he acted as if I had just said I was thinking of ordering soup. All he said was, give it a few days' thought and then if you decide it's not possible I'll have a word with one of my colleagues. A few days later, he asked me, "So, what is it to be? Shall I have a word with someone? Would you like me to get the ball rolling?" And I said, "No, actually. I think I'd like to have this one." And he broke into a smile, and said, "Oh, darling, but that couldn't be better news!" I said, "If you wanted a baby that much, why didn't you just come out and tell me? Why did you put me through this agony?" And all he said was, "That would have been out of the question, because it's your body and your baby and your responsibility and therefore your decision." '

Is this wise or is he just very clever at evading responsibility? Is a woman who is aware of her partner's feelings likely to make a decision to please or displease him instead of thinking about the baby and the responsibilities that this baby implies? Are women more inclined to make decisions 'for' other people because that is what they do most of the time anyway? Do they have to suffer the consequences of a 'considerate' fertility decision before they can trust their own instincts enough to make a decision without a man's support? 'We had no financial constraints,' says Hillary. 'I always expected my husband to support the family. I worked, but it was always piecemeal. I never felt driven.' Although she tried various forms of contraception after giving birth to three children within three years, she 'gradually slipped back into using nothing much at all. You're not having intercourse often, so you think you can afford to take a chance.' She became pregnant again when her youngest was seven and agreed to have an abortion 'largely because my husband did not want more children. He thought it was a lot of work, and that we didn't need another one, that the family was complete. I never went along with him entirely, but I bowed to his views. The abortion went wrong and I was re-admitted to hospital on a stretcher by ambulance, having collapsed and haemorrhaged in the Headmistress' office of my children's school.'

Two years later, she became pregnant again. 'My husband's very first words were, "Whose is it?" and "Get rid of it." I shall remember that forever. I replied, "It's yours, of course," and "No, I shan't get rid of it." He was upset because he was fifty-three and was afraid his friends would laugh at him.' She thinks one of her reasons for getting pregnant again was worry about her fertility. 'I wasn't sure if I hadn't damaged my reproductive parts because I'd had two operations.' When she found out she was pregnant, she thought, 'Wonderful! I can conceive!' Although she worked until the end of the pregnancy, she then spent quite a few years at home playing with her new son, who 'has made my life much more interesting and rewarding'.

Most married women we spoke to had clear ideas about what kind of support they deserved from their husbands – and expressed anger if they didn't receive it. The young and the unattached were much less insistent about their right to support but spoke with great distress about unsympathetic treatment. There were occasional – but persistent – complaints about uninvited lectures on morality from professionals. Many teenagers who had abortions spoke of the decision having been made by their parents. When Tessa became unexpectedly pregnant at sixteen, and her gut feeling was to keep it, she met with opposition not just from her parents but also her grandparents, who were adamantly opposed to a baby outside wedlock.

The baby was not an entire surprise. She and her boyfriend had been 'under pressure of parting. It doesn't sound like much now – it was for two weeks – but it felt like it then.' They had been using condoms, but this time they didn't. There was, she recalls, an 'intuitive feeling . . . a need to fulfil the relationship . . . it seems like a mistake but we probably knew what we were doing.' She took the morning-after pill but it didn't work. 'It's very difficult to make a rational decision as soon as possible.' She went to her doctor, who said a counsellor wouldn't help her, and that she was better off to go straight to the hospital, have the termination, and 'forget about it'.

Initially, her partner couldn't come to terms with it. He said he needed time. Then she started having a lot of pain and was admitted to hospital with a suspected ectopic pregnancy. At the hospital one doctor after another suggested that while they were looking into the ectopic, why didn't they just do a termination? She became so worried that they would do a termination without her permission that in the end she just discharged herself. Still, she wavered about the decision. It was not until sixteen weeks, when she was told it was too late, that she was faced with the decision and decided to have the child.

She went ahead and had the baby and it all worked out well. Not only did the baby make her partner 'pull himself together quickly . . . he had just been mooching around' but it also brought her family together. They rejected it until after they saw it. They had thought of her as a failure because of her A levels, but now she had proven to them that she could 'produce something'. She doesn't think having a baby early has robbed her of her future. Her friends who have had abortions seem, in her opinion, to have a much harder time of it, but with the ones who have gone on to have the babies, she has seen 'good qualities develop'. They are 'less wild, more fulfilled'. What she regrets most of all is how little support she got when she was pregnant. The abortion counselling she did have was helpful, but it ended when she decided to keep the child. She now thinks that it was after that decision that she needed support and guidance more than ever. The decision itself was straightforward: 'Having babies is one of those things when you go with your feelings.'

But what happens to your feelings when you must confront statistics? This is fast becoming a universal experience as more and more women undergo genetic screening.

'How was I supposed to make a responsible decision?' says Belinda. She was offered an amniocentesis during her third pregnancy on account of being in her late thirties. 'Just put yourself in my shoes. There you are, sitting in a hospital with your friendly genetic counsellor. There, in the mound in front of you, is this baby who is clearly just one person. Who is either defective or not defective. You are afraid of its being defective, but how afraid? So afraid that you are not too afraid to run a one per cent risk of losing the baby as a direct result of an invasive test? If you are so afraid that you are not afraid of a one per cent risk, does that mean that the baby is one per cent unwanted? There is no such thing, of course! The only sane course is to weigh the one per cent risk against the risk of a defect. But that's not so easy either. Because, as any good counsellor will tell you, the word defect is a blanket term. Some children born with Down's syndrome are less seriously affected than others. Some can attend normal schools and function independently. In France, where they monitor vitamin and hormonal deficiencies more carefully than they do in the UK, they claim to get better results. Furthermore, many parents of Down's children speak of how lovable they are, and how rewarding it has been to look after them. How are you meant to measure these unquantifiable arguments against the rows of large figures? Short answer: you can't. Or rather, all you can say is, can I accept a handicapped child? Will I be able to care for it? But if you start thinking in these terms, it is easy to start taking a low probability for a certainty. After all, the risk of a defect for your age group is two per cent, while the risk of a defect according to the results of a newer, better blood test is 0.1 per cent – although the accuracy of this test is somewhat in doubt because it very much depends on being able to pinpoint the date of conception, which happens to be something you're not altogether sure about. So let's stand back a bit. Let's take note of the fact that the blood test result is not just a little, but a lot better than the other indicator. The blood test indicates that there is a one in a thousand chance of a defective baby. But how to bridge the gap between a thousand imaginary babies and one real one?'

Her point was that no decision she took could possibly be rational. 'It was just a case of closing my eyes and jumping, figuring out what scenario I could live with least. The only thing that saved me was that I didn't have to share the decision with anyone else. That way would have been madness.' Her words were echoed by many other women who found themselves in similar situations – as well as one woman who found herself way, way beyond the reach of normal genetic counselling. We would like to quote her here – not because anyone reading this book is likely ever to be in the same position, but because of the way she describes the strange interplay of the intellectual and the emotional in the formation of her decision, and also because of the troubling issues she raises about choice, control, and the possible consequences of joint decision-making.

Valerie first tried for a child when she was in her mid-thirties – only to discover that she had 'horrendous' fertility problems on account of an IUD she had when she was a teenager. Although she eventually got pregnant, her son was born three months early. There was nothing wrong with him – they told her it was a 'problem with the pregnancy': in other words, the problem was her body. Because of her history, she 'thought it couldn't happen again. I didn't want to wait long if I was going to have another, because I was thirty-nine, but at the same time I wasn't ready, he was still so tiny, so in itself it was madness to find myself pregnant again when he was six months old. But anyway it happened. And in fact they were triplets.'

By chance, she found out about a new procedure, which was 'neither legal nor illegal', which permitted for a partial abortion. 'I must have read an article, or talked to my sister-in-law who has twins. It all happened by accident, by pure chance. When I first thought about it, I thought it was infinitely preferable to letting nature take its course. The chances of a pregnancy reaching term are much lower for twins, are even lower for triplets, but in my case, with my history, the consensus among three or four consultants was that given my age, given the history, triplets would be a lot higher risk than for someone else . . . the doctors felt that since I'd had one premature baby. But this is what I was saying, about running into medical matters when you have all the information to hand and it's a totally grey area, making a decision to have a partial abortion that carried a risk of destroying the entire pregnancy. They were all healthy, it was a terrible thing to do, it was a ghastly thing to do, they could all have possibly survived. . . . I had a lot of doctors helping me make the decision, but they all disagreed. The people who had been involved in our fertility treatment just couldn't accept it. They also knew in my case I wasn't likely to get pregnant again. My consultant here wouldn't touch it. The man who did it is very courageous. I made the final decision by myself. The doctors wouldn't decide because they all felt it was an area well beyond normal medicine, and it goes into realms of your own feelings far beyond. I respected that but found it very frightening because I didn't have any guidance . . . I didn't have any knowledge of what they might do. . . .'

But it seemed like a 'way out'. 'It seemed like a compromise to all the other options, like losing all three, or having the triplets and not being able to care for them. We even discussed having the triplets and then having one adopted, and then we realised that was a madness. We considered every solution. I thought adoption would be better than destroying the fetus. I have always been in favour of abortion, but then when you are faced with the problem yourself . . . I talked to a friend who had had several abortions. I couldn't understand why I was making such a fuss, especially since I wasn't giving up a pregnancy, because what you're actually doing is preserving life, in theory, not just destroying . . . but I had been working so hard to have children, and then this. . . .

'I didn't know if the procedure was successful until after they were born. I had a ten day period after the operation when I was just thinking, what had I done? It was hell. I was all alone because my husband and my son were away on holiday. The holiday was already booked, and we should all have gone together, and so I thought, why spoil everybody's fun? We did the right thing in that we have healthy twin daughters, but I'll have deep regrets until the day I die and I'm not sure about the one that I lost.

'That said, I would do the same again. I don't think I would have had the courage to carry on with the pregnancy, because it would have been even more scary, and that was the risk we took, that was what we discussed, the knowledge that by doing that, if anything had gone wrong, it could have been totally unrelated to what I had done, but we would probably have had a sense of guilt. Nobody could have ever proved it. The doctors warned us about this. . . . I have never felt more in control. It was very scary and I was very alone. And I think women who argue about this business of being in control do not understand what they're saying, actually. They think in ideal terms, but it's a partnership, and in situations like that, that involve moral and ethical dilemmas, ethically some of the doctors wiped their hands of it, not because they were anti-abortion, but because this particular procedure was a different ballgame, and you are totally alone. You are in control as far as anybody can be. Some women who talk about it as an ideal don't understand the implications of being in control, of the arguments they are making . . .

'I mean, I was given information that I didn't want to have. There were equations all over the paper. I sat down with the doctor and said, OK, if I did this, this, and this. . . . He offered me hundreds of alternatives. I mean, I decided not to have an amnio because that would have been in itself a high risk of miscarriage. "For example," he said, "the chances of having a genetically defective child are quite high for someone in your age bracket, and with three your chances are much higher." And I said, "What happens if you destroy one, and of the two that are born, one is genetically defective?" and he said, "OK, I'll do an amnio on the three," and I said, "What's the risk?" and he said, "Quite high," and I thought for ten minutes, and said "No way" . . .'

She doesn't remember the exact moment when she made her decision. She was always leaning in that direction, and when her husband left on holiday, 'he knew it was likely'. 'I just thought in terms of health, in terms of pressure on us as a family, I just couldn't imagine. I think it was quite a detached decision, I had to be detached. I had to try and put away the emotions. I literally weighed the emotions up against the intellectual arguments, and these were all options, so it was probably more intellectual. There were some indications that it was the right thing to do, probably intellectually it was the right thing to do, probably emotionally not necessarily at all, but funnily enough, because you're still pregnant afterwards, you don't feel any different about the intervention, there's no practical sign of it at all, you don't imagine it hits you after your babies are born. You suddenly realise there could have been another one there, and that feeling has gone on, that feeling of loss. The better the twins do, the worse it makes it, though it would seem more logical the other way around. In a way that's ultimately why I urged my husband to go away on holiday, because I thought, well, if I'm going to carry the responsibility . . . Actually, it wasn't just me carrying the responsibility, but in the end it was largely me. I don't even want him to feel that he influenced me, and I was desperately lonely, but in the end I think you live with it much better if you've done that. I didn't want . . . I suppose what I wanted to avoid most was ghastliness between us. I felt if it had been a totally joint decision, there's always the possibility of a disagreement or some kind of anger or accusation afterwards. He knew everything that was going on, and we had discussed it, and I asked him to trust me to make the best decision and that seemed the best thing to do. . . . He was distressed but he knew I was doing what I felt was right.'

In other words, she believes she saved her marriage by taking ultimate responsibility for the decision. But it is also worth noting that she only did so after asking for and getting his blessing for this course of action. Here, as elsewhere, a curious game seems to have to occur. The man must offer to give up his right to take part in the decision for the woman to proceed with any peace of mind. The woman must not insist on her right to final say without first consulting with the man and asking for his permission to act alone. At the same time there is an eerie sense that the decision was really made before the discussion even began – a gut decision in response to the woman's greatest fear – about her body, about her ability to look after children properly, about social disgrace, about making an irreversible decision to have an abortion. In this light, the discussion is a testing of that gut decision. If a woman is single and making a decision on her own, she'll often set a capricious-sounding test for herself. If it's not placing a bet on the Grand National, she'll find some other way of at least half-convincing herself that the decision is really out of her hands, or already written in the sky, that someone out there has approved the course of action she is considering. If a woman is making a decision with a partner, the discussion is an elaborate dance she performs for permission to follow her instincts. If such a minuet does not occur, trust is destroyed – sometimes irretrievably. If either party feels tricked or intimidated or emotionally blackmailed or taken for granted or even unconsulted, the resentment – whether it is spoken or unspoken – is huge and can have terrible consequences. Because it is so often the woman who makes the final decision, it is just as often the man who feels betrayed. All too often, the confused and arbitrary decision sets the stage for a new drama that has the inevitable sound of a classic tragedy.

'I was overcome with such sadness,' says Ramu of his wife's quickly implemented abortion. 'It was half mine but she never gave me a chance to consider the idea. I know I ought to have said something, but what? I felt so powerless and I couldn't even tell her about my sadness, so we drifted apart.' Six months later, he had a serious affair and he and his wife parted. It was only a year after that, when they got together again, that he was able to express his feelings to her.

Says Miles of his lover's unnegotiated pregnancy, 'I suspected that her motive was to involve me in some kind of permanent relationship. But it hasn't worked out that way. I could never live with a person who behaved that deviously.'

Says Gerald of his wife's second pregnancy, 'I'll always remember the little circle in the test tube of the pregnancy test. For me, it meant prison. That was the last straw. I knew I would stay home and be the father of my children, but it was over between us. She could have my body but not my soul. From then on, I took my affections elsewhere. I knew it was just a matter of time before we split up.'

CHAPTER EIGHT

THE FINAL SOLUTION

'You want to know why I don't want a vasectomy?' says Peter. 'I'll tell you why I don't want a vasectomy. I don't want a vasectomy (a) because I believe it's a procedure that can cause you serious harm (b) because I dislike surgical procedures in general, and (c) because I don't want a vasectomy. That accounts for (d) (e) and (f) as well.'

Although vasectomy is fast becoming one of the most popular forms of birth control in this country, it remains a source of dread to the uninitiated. 'I was playing around with the idea,' says one man who has three surprise children and five abortions to his credit. 'So I went to the doctor. He turned out to be a louche sort of character in a shiny dark suit. After he had me drop my trousers, he gave me a flashy, sinister smile that was like something out of a Roald Dahl book, and I decided, no way! And that was that. Later I also thought, in this AIDS environment, I'm not even promiscuous any more, so why go to all that bother?'

Other men we spoke to cited friends as cautionary examples. One knew someone whose operation had gone wrong. 'He was swollen, and in excruciating pain, for months.' Another knew someone who had had 'the chop' because he had decided that his four children had ruined his life – only to change his mind after meeting someone new and realising it was his wife who had ruined his life, not his children. Now he was desolate that he could not give his new love the child she deserved.

'I'd like to keep my options open.' This is the stock response men give for not getting sterilised even when they are serious about not wanting any more children. For women, too, it is the distant prospect of 'something' happening to their husbands and children, and the subsequent necessity to 'start again', that put so many off the idea of tubal ligation. You get the impression, however, that unless 'something else' happens to jolt them out of lethargy, or 'someone else' takes the initiative, it will never happen. 'Really my husband must go and get sterilised,' says Frances. 'I considered sterilisation myself but I don't think I could. They tried to talk me into it after my second for medical reasons, and I'm glad I didn't, obviously, because that would have meant no third child. Now I think it's not worth it. My fertility must be on the wane now in a big way. . . . I suppose I have always assumed that it's men who get sterilised. The only time it comes up is when I go to the doctors and pick up a leaflet and then it falls under the bed to join all the old diaphragms. . . .'

You see the same type of reluctance in couples who insist they have no children 'by conscious choice'. Fiona and Richard had gone into marriage assuming children would turn up eventually, but they found themselves postponing the decision over and over. A scare made them realise that, in fact, they both dreaded the prospect. After that, Fiona suggested that she be sterilised, 'but Richard was unsure whether he might not perhaps resent me for the finality of it, but now that he is older I know that he, too, is relieved not to have children. He is reluctant (and too squeamish) to have a vasectomy and I would not insist for my sake. We have tried the pill, and the dutch cap: I had problems with the cap, and the FPA had to try different varieties for me, but I was never really happy. We settled for condoms for a while but didn't like the smell, the feel, and the loss of momentum at the peak of excitement. I am now on the minipill and again seriously considering sterilisation, and yet . . . and yet . . . There is always that niggling feeling of finality. Will I again feel that I have cheated my last chance to be a mum, and have I cheated Richard?'

If you talk to people who have had the procedure done, however, there is seldom a sense that they are wavering in a sea of hellish 'what if' questions. Most describe their decision either as a necessary and fitting curbing of natural urges, or else as the lesser of two evils. A number of younger women we spoke to, who had had several pregnancies in rapid succession, talked about their bodies as if they were beasts that needed taming. Sterilisation spelled relief for them, and for women who felt they had gone over their natural allotment, it meant the end of a compulsive habit. 'I know I could have gone on and on,' says Roxanne, who had four children when she booked in for a sterilisation, and five children by the time she finally had it done. 'Although I have always had very bad pregnancies, babies give me great pleasure and a sense of purpose. I went into a very bad depression after my second, for example. It was only when I had another one that I began to come out of it. But a time arrived when I had to consider the needs of the other members of the family.' Anna also discussed her decision as a belated form of selflessness. After her fourth child, she was beginning to feel embarrassed – and be teased – about her 'greedy urge' to reproduce. And so, when her doctor gave her a 'gentle talk' about the world population problems (and this type of intervention does happen) she agreed to be sterilised. 'I know the family has benefited materially because of it. Neither hubby nor I had high-paying jobs – he was working at a garage and I was working as a waitress and we were just getting to the stage when all the children were starting to want things their friends had that we could not afford because of our food bills. If I hadn't been sterilised, I know I would not have been able to stop having children.'

Dorothy also sees her entire family as having benefited from her decision to be sterilised. The alternative would have been to live in fear of mental breakdown. 'I have two normal healthy daughters, both planned,' she says. 'The first pregnancy was dominated by continuous nausea and sickness throughout and ended in a forceps delivery.' She was also grieving for her father, who had died two months into the pregnancy. 'The second pregnancy was similar to the first, but the birth was normal. I was severely depressed during the pregnancy, and so high after the birth that I had to be sedated five or six days afterwards. Then, four or five months later, we moved house. After that I became severely depressed. I can't remember exactly, but I think I tried to commit suicide. I was then committed to a mental home, where I received electric shock treatment. I had no desire to have more children – we had agreed on an intended family size of two children. I am not a particularly maternal person, and my husband and doctor were worried as it seemed I was at risk of having another. My GP thought it would be the end of me. It was quite obvious to me that it was I who wanted to have more children, not my husband. I think it was a sensible conclusion to come to. My husband has never entertained the use of condoms, and I wasn't keen on the pill. Life has been much better since I was sterilised. It's enabled me to lead a normal sex life without fear of pregnancy.'

That, after all, is the goal that sterilisation is meant to achieve. But here she describes the fear of mental illness as the reason, and the convenience as a happy end result. However they feel about the procedure afterwards, most people seem to have it done for personal reasons, or to achieve a clear and immediate goal. 'I just loved having babies,' says Carla, 'and so I kept having them, one after the other. It was when I was pregnant for the fifth time that I began to see that there were problems in my marriage and that my husband might leave me if I carried on with the pregnancy. I went and asked for an abortion, but my doctor said, no, go ahead with this one and then we'll have you sterilised. And that's what I did. I felt sad afterwards, as if part of my life were over, as indeed it was, but then I moved on to new things, a new chapter of my life began – although I did not get what I thought I wanted at the time, which was to keep my husband. I did it for him, but it didn't work.' Another thing that doesn't seem to work is to avoid having to be sterilised by asking your partner to be sterilised instead. As one man told us, 'My wife doubted herself because she had been told she couldn't have another child. And so my theory is she wanted to make sure I was as damaged as she was. Oh, and of course, it was a way of keeping me from wandering off and having children with someone else. Well, as I told her at the time, I would rather do without sex altogether than agree to her request.'

If the motive behind such a request is selfishness or convenience, it is usually rejected. The exception is when there has been a surprise pregnancy after the family has been deemed complete, followed by an upsetting abortion. Two children, one abortion, and then a vasectomy is a common pattern. 'It was a joint decision. It was a way of sharing the hurt,' says Karen of her husband's vasectomy. They had been discussing the possibility of one of them being sterilised in a desultory manner, until a faulty condom resulted in an unplanned pregnancy and an abortion. 'Up until that point I would have considered sterilisation but, after that, I decided it was his turn to do something to his body. I think the reason most men won't consider vasectomy is that they are so attached to their members that they can't bear anyone touching it for any reason other than their pleasure. If you ask me, vasectomies aren't painful enough. They should last at least as long as labour.'

She is not the only woman to sound vindictive about her husband's sterilisation. 'You want to have a voice in the decisions?' many women seem to be saying. 'Fine, then start by sharing the hurt. You mutilate yourself for a change. *You* make an irreversible decision, and I'll watch.'

CHAPTER NINE

WHEN NATURE HAS THE LAST LAUGH: UNPLANNED INFERTILITY

There is no one more serene, more apparently in control, than the mature adult who has decided not to have children. It doesn't matter what the exact reason is: underpinning it will be the sense that this person knows exactly what he or she wants out of life, exactly what are the necessary components of happiness and fulfilment. There is a sense of destiny, a certainty that the world will look just the same in ten years' time as it looks today.

There is no one more confused, more stripped of power, than the mature adult who runs into fertility trouble. 'First I didn't know what to think,' says one young woman of her failure to conceive on demand. 'All my life, I had been trying *not* to have a baby. I thought a baby would simply appear because we had expressed the desire. I know it sounds ridiculous – like I thought I was living in an enchanted castle. Of course I knew the facts of life, but emotionally it was as if I believed eggs were fertilised by wishes. After about three months of failure, I sneaked into a bookstore and looked up fertility. I remember being very worried that the people around me would see what I was reading and know my problem. Anyway, it was in this way that I discovered I was probably only fertile for less than twenty-four hours during a cycle. No one had ever told me that before! I felt cheated.

'I imagine many women would panic at this point, especially if they thought they didn't have many years left. I was twenty-five at the time, so my feelings were perhaps atypical. I didn't panic. I just took my failure to conceive as evidence that there was something wrong with my body. This was a thought that had plagued me during pre-adolescence, so much so that when my periods started, at fifteen, I almost didn't believe it. My self-doubt was stronger than the reality. Now, once again, I was too ashamed about my body's failures to discuss them with anyone, and that included my husband and my friends as well as doctors. If I saw an article about pregnancy or babies in the paper, I would be overcome with grief and on several occasions I went so far as to cut the offending page out of the paper so that my husband wouldn't see it.

'Every time I had a period I felt this sense of failure all the more keenly. Then as the cycle progressed, I would entertain vain hopes. I would monitor my barren body for signs of change. Sore breasts, fatigue, nausea, I detected them all until another furtive trip to a bookstore led me to a passage on hysterical pregnancy. After a year, I went to a doctor, who told me to keep temperature charts and have sex more often. I'm told now that such charts are useless for timing conception, but three months later I did succeed in getting pregnant. By that time I was not so much desperate as determined – my husband, who had been working on a rig in the North Sea, was about to take a job in Iraq. I knew that if I got pregnant before he accepted, he would say no to the job. And I was right. I know it's silly to say this, but I'm convinced that until I had that objective, which I saw as larger and more important than myself, my fears about my body were keeping me from ovulating.

'I also remember what a relief it was – just before all this happened – to meet another infertile couple. I no longer felt singled out. I borrowed a book from them and still had it when I found out I was pregnant. This other couple did not take my good news well. It did not seem fair, as this other woman was far more maternal than I was. Shortly thereafter, I had a threatened miscarriage, and my doubts about my body returned with a vengeance, even though it went to term and resulted in a healthy birth.'

Shock, denial, grief, shame, a sharp drop in self-confidence, the conviction that you have been singled out, and sometimes even the suspicion that you are being punished. These are the feelings reported by women who suffer from unplanned infertility – by

When Nature Has the Last Laugh

which we mean, women who have had miscarriages or stillbirths or find they cannot conceive according to schedule – even if they have had children before. For many, it is the first indication that the body does not always obey the will. If that person's strategy has always been to live by strictly imposed, carefully rational planning, the failure to conceive can challenge an entire way of life.

That said, there is no predicting how an individual will react to the news of fertility trouble. It is almost the other way round – your emotional response is the real news. You only find out how important the ability to have children is to you as and when fertility problems become apparent.

'When I was told I was pregnant after a faulty test,' says Margaret, 'I was devastated. This really brought home to me my real feelings. We talked, we discussed it, we tried to come to terms with it, and eventually a week later started to accept that it was meant to be. Never did I consider abortion for my own convenience. However my doctor finally assured me that it was a false result and that I was not after all pregnant. Oh, the fickleness of the human mind! I felt cheated and every bit as depressed as I had been when I thought I was, when I found that I wasn't!'

People who have gone in for fertility treatment speak of their experience in the same strong words. Their stories are all about power, or rather the stripping away of power. There is always a sense of being a social outcast. As one woman told us, 'When I found out we couldn't have children, my first thought was, now I know what it's like to be gay, what it's like to be excluded from normal life.'

Not everyone feels such a sense of tragedy. Women who have serious misgivings about childbearing or childrearing often take the first indication of infertility as an invitation to give up. 'I laughed,' said Blanche. 'All I could think was, all those years of wasted contraceptive effort. I needn't have bothered!' For women who attempt parenthood out of a sense of obligation – because it is something one *should* try, or because one's partner has expressed a desire for children – one single sign from on high that they might be infertile is enough to justify a decision to stop trying. This kind of fatalism is evident in the reluctant potential parent even when she is an agnostic in all other matters, even when she is the type of person always to go for a second opinion.

If a woman is fairly confident about her body, but has mixed feelings about having a child, the failure to produce a child can be a relief. Melanie, for example, had been in two minds about having a third child. When the question took on an extra urgency after a friend the same age became pregnant with a third child she described as her 'last chance', Melanie decided that she 'ought to at least try and see if it might be possible'. She was 'very pleased' when she found out that she was pregnant, but not at all upset when she lost the baby at three months. Having entered into pregnancy half out of a desire for a child, and half out of a feeling that a third child was something she ought to try for, she took the miscarriage as a 'sign from the gods . . . in a way I was relieved. I said to myself, "I've done my bit. I don't have to try again." '

Again, we see a woman taking comfort from the certainty of the uncertainty factor. Some decisions are in her hands; some are not. That stoical feeling seems only to be possible if the powers that be are invisible. The moment the power is seen to be invested in doctors, the story changes, as we see in this account of a missed abortion (a fetal death that does not result in an immediate miscarriage):

'They discovered the problem when I went in for a routine scan. They couldn't find a fetal heartbeat. They brought in extra doctors and peered into the screen for a full twenty minutes before they bothered to tell me what was going on, but of course it was clear to me way before then that there was something very wrong. They told me I had to go straight to another hospital for the "evacuation of the products of conception". I had to go downstairs to the maternity ward to use the telephone to make arrangements for the night for my other children. Next to the phone was an advertisement for "baby's first picture". I was having to speak to a number of mothers I didn't know very well. I didn't want to tell them what had happened but it was very difficult to keep my voice steady. Then I had to go up to genetic screening again, where they made me wait in a room with all the other pregnant women waiting for their scans. I alternated between extreme jealousy – why did it have to be me, why were all these other women so much luckier – and extreme worry that I was going to break into tears and upset them when they were probably already very nervous. This same awkwardness existed in the hospital ward where I soon found myself, as half the patients there were miscarriages and the other half were terminations.

'By then I had become convinced that it had all been a mistake. I wanted proof, but apparently this was all part of the process of grieving – denial, in other words. The nurses were very kind and took turns sitting down with me, but their fatalistic reassurances about how it was all meant to be hit me the wrong way. I felt they were saying, "It's all out of our hands, too, we must follow the doctor's orders." Even as I was wheeled into the operating room, I was convinced – partly because there had been no bleeding – that they were taking my living baby away from me. I know in my sane mind that isn't so, but that was how I continued to feel, robbed of my baby, and duped into going along with doctors' orders.'

A woman's body, a baby's life – these are phrases that people debating fertility throw about like confetti. But in the context we are looking at now, what do they really mean? In the preceding account, the fetus was dead and the woman's body needed and got efficient emergency treatment and was back to normal a few days later. The doctors did what they were there to do; the nurses could not be accused of ignoring her feelings. Even so, the woman describes the experience as shaming – she has failed to perform like a proper woman – and as a usurping of her power: once she was in hospital, the doctors took over and she was unable to influence events even when she became convinced that there must have been a mistake.

Her words are echoed by many a woman undergoing IVF – especially the ones who do not succeed in getting pregnant. 'I know they meant well, but they treated my body as if it were a box of cornflakes,' says one woman who now has two healthy children courtesy of this technology. Almost all the people we spoke to who had undergone fertility treatment, even the ones who were ultimately glad to have availed themselves of these services, complained of medical affronts:

'I had to have two semen tests,' one man told us. 'For some reason they involved two different hospitals. At the first hospital they gave me a sample jar and sent me home and told me to bring in the sample as soon as I produced it. That was bad enough, having to masturbate into a jar and then call a minicab. But the second time was even worse. It was in the basement. I went and asked for my sample jar and they looked at me and said, "What are you on about? No, you're going to have to do it here." "Where?" I asked. They pointed me in the direction of the toilet, which was occupied. Also in the queue was a rather large woman who was there to do a urine sample. When my turn came, I found I couldn't produce. And so I had to go out and beg the people at the desk to be able to take the jar home. "I'll bring it right back," I said "I promise!" They thought about it for a while and then they said, "Well all right, just this once. So long as you realise you're forcing us to break the rules." '

His sperm, he assured us, turned out to be perfectly fine. But when another man we spoke to went through the same tests, and it emerged that he had a low sperm count, their doctor saw nothing wrong in giving the bad news to his wife when he wasn't present. Another insensitive comment by another insensitive doctor, this time to a wife about the results of a sperm–mucus compatibility test: 'You seem to be killing off your husband's sperm.'

'Just relax!' fertility patients are always being told. What many of them ask is: how? All too often fertility clinics run simultaneously with and use the same waiting rooms as antenatal clinics; meetings for the sub-fertile are held in the parent craft room; patients who have determined that they will be ovulating on a Wednesday are told that that's no good, that doesn't fit in with their schedule, as the clinic only offers ultrasound on Thursdays. Many clinics do not offer continuous care, with the inevitable resulting record-keeping errors, and there are too many stories about doctors who ought to know better passing on gratuitous and incorrect advice about the correct positions and timing for procreative intercourse.

And then there are the various controversies that patients will find themselves exacerbating without ever even realising. There is, for example, a controversy about keeping temperature charts to determine ovulations. Some doctors feel so strongly that they are not worth the effort that they have been known to tear them up in front of their patients. While this may be liberating to some temperature-takers, it is distressing to others. Other patients talk of a similar confusion after switching from a doctor who believes stress is related to infertility, to a doctor who has doubts. 'It was wonderful,' as one man recalls. 'He leaned over to me and bellowed, "Get this into your head! *Stress causes impotence, not infertility!*" His bedside manner did wonders for my sex life.'

Even those patients who receive the most considerate of treatment show signs of emotional scarring. People whose fertility problem goes undiagnosed and people who have had their tubes cleared to no avail, or undergone unsuccessful IVF or GIFT treatment, describe themselves as worthless, defective, evolutionary mistakes. Sometimes there is a bitter search for causes. Because infertility is frequently iatrogenic, in other words, caused by previous medical procedures, this will often turn into anger against the medical establishment. But, just as often, the searcher will turn the sword against herself. 'This is happening because of my own stupidity, because I had that late abortion/took the pill for too many years/didn't bother to find out the side-effects of the IUD before having one put in.' Superstition makes a big comeback: 'I'm convinced it happened because I was too sure things were finally working out,' says one woman whose third IVF treatment resulted in a pregnancy that ended in stillbirth at twenty-two weeks. 'The day before it happened I had been on a shopping spree for baby things. It's very dangerous to count your chickens before they've hatched.' It's surprising how often people explain new difficulties as retribution for old transgressions. Here's a typically offhand comment from a woman who was just about to go into hospital for her first delivery – of twins – at age thirty-nine: 'It's strange wanting them so much after all those abortions for all those years. Our friends tell us we're having twins because we're being punished.'

Says another woman of her state of mind when she became pregnant three months after a miscarriage: 'I couldn't trust my body. I thought it was out to get me, to punish me for all the things I had done to it. And so I expected to miscarry at any moment. When I did have a threatened miscarriage at ten weeks, I'm afraid my first thought was not, "Oh, the baby." It was, "What is wrong with me? Why can't I do this any more?" It was only when I went in for an emergency ultrasound, and saw the fetus, who didn't just have a beating heart, but was whirling around the womb, having a wonderful time, that I remembered what all this was really about. Not just me, but that little creature as well. It had no idea how defective its mother was, and, you know? it didn't seem to matter. After that, every time I had doubts about myself, I cheered myself up by remembering that picture.'

In other words, the drama of public failure came to an abrupt end with the sight of a healthy fetus bouncing around the ultrasound screen. It was only when she had 'living proof' that she began to visualise the pregnancy differently. It was not just the story of a recalcitrant, rebellious body. Inside that drama was another drama that was beginning, very literally, to take on a life of its own, and, to use the woman's own words, 'it was better than any baby I could possibly have imagined.'

But until such a time as a woman has that living proof, and by this we mean not simply proof of existence, but a visual proof, proof of a separate and particular and unique existence that does not fit exactly with the fantasy baby, her feelings about a pregnancy will be dominated by her feelings about her body, or rather, her feelings about the history of her body. This will be largely because her body is real to her while the baby is not: no amount of enforced compassion can change this. In fact, sentimentalising about fetal rights and futures is bound only to make the fantasy baby into more of a fantasy than ever. The body, meanwhile, continues to be judged strictly according to its performance record, as we see in this account by a woman who has had repeated difficulties:

'We were married in 1983, when I was twenty-six and Simon was thirty-five. In 1985 we decided to start a family. In May 1986 I had a missed abortion at thirteen weeks, followed by a D and C. We were devastated. Naïvely I thought that sort of thing didn't happen to me. Happily, I conceived within a few months but there were many problems with that pregnancy. I was resting and bleeding for ages in hospital (including over Christmas) with a placenta praevia, before going into premature labour at twenty-one weeks. Needless to say the baby did not survive. . . . It was a ghastly experience, and for quite a while we put the baby question on hold. We felt our lives had been so disrupted – we couldn't plan holidays or generally do anything. Should we move? Could we afford to? – all silly things like do we decorate or buy new carpets?

'In 1988 I gave up my full-time job and began to work from home, part-time, setting up my own small business. . . . We weren't really trying for a baby and did not feel desperate but I had a laparoscopy and dye in May 1990 to rule out any problems. We had also done a post-coital test which revealed that sperm count and compatibility were OK. In July 1991 I conceived again. But this was an ectopic pregnancy and I had major surgery in August that year. For the fourth time I became pregnant at the end of November 1991 but, again, I lost it in December at eight weeks. This time it was a spontaneous abortion. As you can imagine, by now, we were beginning to feel that fate was against us. My point in telling you all this is we feel although we decided to have a family as far back as I can remember, we still haven't achieved it! I've read many books on all subjects connected with pregnancy, childbirth, parenthood, and none cover any of my experiences. There are repeated miscarriages – usually hormonal or due to problems with the cervix – or complete fertility problems. Nobody seems to cater for someone like me who is just working through the book and trying some new problem every time!'

At the time of her letter, she was pregnant again, and doing well at twenty-four weeks. Although they were feeling very positive, she said, 'We have decided that if things don't work out this time we won't try again. We have both had a lot of emotional problems to contend with. . . . Everyone tells me I could go on but to be honest, I've had enough. My determination used to be a lot greater than it is now and I'm running out of perseverance.'

And that is the rule: no matter how well things are going, you take your history with you. This woman has good and specific reasons to have shaky confidence in her ability to reproduce: it is only by producing a healthy baby that her feelings about her body will change. And even with success, doubts can persevere – and affect later fertility decisions. Caroline, for example, had to go through two years of infertility treatment before she managed to conceive. 'You can't help feeling you are less than female. And your faith in your body continues to decline. The longer the treatment, the more serious the tests.' Although she did end up having a child who is now perfectly healthy, she remained convinced there was something wrong with her body because the baby was born nine weeks premature. She was certain, therefore, that she would never be able to conceive again, and so did not pay much attention to contraception. Before the baby was even out of the neonatal ward, she conceived again. For her, as for so many women, the label of sub-fertile or infertility does not come easily unstuck.

The verdicts such women pass on themselves have a primitive ring to them. 'GIFT didn't work on me because my eggs are bad,' one woman informed us. 'Because of the preparations they did in the lab, the sperm were perfect. It was my fault I miscarried at seven weeks.'

A lot of rewriting goes on. 'I thought I was fertile. Now that I know I'm not, my whole life seems a mockery.' 'I thought I had received good sex education. Now I realise I was brainwashed into relying on contraceptives that have ruined my body.' 'They told me there was nothing wrong with the fetus, that it was something wrong with the pregnancy, in other words, me.'

Perhaps most important is the way in which a woman's medical history affects the way she makes decisions. 'Before I had my first child at thirty-seven, I had had several miscarriages,' says Winny. 'And so when they offered me an amniocentesis with a one per cent chance of miscarriage, I said no way. I want that child, whatever it's like, and I'm not sure I can carry a baby to term in the best of circumstances. I can't afford to take any risks. When I got pregnant a year later, though, I felt differently, even though the risks of a Down's child were not that much greater. It's just that I could live with the risk factor, because I felt more confident. I knew I could produce a child.' For other women, self-doubt persists despite evidence to the contrary. There are many women with three or four children who persist in thinking of themselves as sub-fertile. Likewise, a woman who has undergone fertility treatment is likely to use contraception erratically even after she has had a child, even if she's not ready yet for another. She is also likely to want to dispense with contraception altogether because she mistrusts it so – women who have suffered fertility problems are some of the most likely candidates for natural family planning. Even if such a woman learns her lessons well and conceives very quickly for the second time, she will often continue to discuss her body as if it were a box marked 'This way up – fragile'. And the terrible thing is, no one else seems to realise. Hailey, for example, has a long and terrible history including miscarriages, stillbirths, an ectopic pregnancy, and ovarian cysts, many of which misfortunes she attributes to an early illegal abortion. She is now forty-eight and childless. When she was confronted with the prospect of having one of her ovaries removed, to spare her the possibility of eventual cancer, she was terribly distressed, not because it lowered the chances of having a child, but because the removal of an ovary would leave her feeling damaged and incomplete. Eve, a fifty-year-old mother of three who has also had two miscarriages and an abortion, reports a similar affront: 'I had an argument when I went in for a repair of a vaginal prolapse. The registrar said they might as well take out the whole works so that I had no risk of uterine or ovarian cancer in ten years. And I said, "I'll sign the paper so long as you agree to take off my left little finger." "Why?" he asked. "Because," I said, "it is as useless as my uterus or ovaries." Luckily I didn't have to go through with it. I would feel deformed without it.'

Again, and again, and again, the preoccupation has to do with the body, or rather, what is wrong with the body, and this syndrome is inadvertently exacerbated when the people around the woman have a utilitarian understanding of fertility. It is often said, for example, that it is important for the woman who has had a stillbirth to be able to see and hold her dead child, as this aids in the grieving process. This may be so, but the women we spoke to who had suffered this misfortune complain routinely about insensitive treatment even where their feelings about the baby are respected. We would suggest that this is because many of their other feelings are left unacknowledged and so easily stepped on. Because they are grieving for the baby *and* their body. Their body has failed them and their children: they can no longer think of themselves as fertile, until such a time as there is proof to the contrary. As one woman who suffered a stillbirth told us, 'They kept on saying, "Oh don't worry, you're young. You could have another one within the year." They didn't seem to realise that that was not the issue.'

You are only as good, it seems, as your last conception. To quote Marilyn, who has three children by her first marriage, but who has been unable to conceive in her second marriage, 'People keep telling me, "Well at least you have the others to console you, it's not as bad as it would be if you didn't have any kids at all." But the truth is, I am totally devastated. My idea of my body has been exposed as false. I had always been so confident of my power to conceive. And now it just isn't there. It's like driving down a busy road and having your engine cut out. How can you ever trust that engine again?'

Some people adjust to the idea that children might not be forthcoming. Having decided that they're not up to the expense and/or trauma of treatment, they agree 'to let nature take its course and see what happens. . . . That way there's not the same sense of failure.' But for those who do continue to 'try', each unwanted period brings new grief and a new challenge to sexual identity. 'Every time I saw a woman with a baby, I thought: "Why is she so lucky? What did she do to deserve such happiness? Why am I the one who has to suffer? What is wrong with me? What did I do to deserve this fate?"' Then there are the technical problems: 'Intercourse became a duty, no – something even worse than that. Something terribly urgent, like mouth-to-mouth resuscitation. I would get one of the signs and phone him at work. . . . I'd say to him, "Get home at once or else . . ." It was as if I were in the emergency room of a hospital. It was no way to live.

'I never even knew I wanted children until I found out I couldn't. So naturally I wondered if I had taken leave of my senses.' It is in this spirit of defeat and self-questioning that most couples finally seek medical advice. They are at their most suggestible. Having lost their old version of events, they are receptive to – and even eager for – a new version. They are likely to put too much trust in their doctors, casting them as saviours. This happens even when the fertility problem is the result of a previous medical intervention. Some doctors have been known to exploit this trust: Sheila Kitzinger has complained that fertility doctors seem to take personal credit for the babies they make possible. (In one famous case in the US, the doctor turned out to be his programme's main sperm donor.) She also complains that patients are unaware of the low chances of success of a given treatment.[1] It is also true, however, that desperate people who think of their bodies as defective will grasp at straws. They will want to think of their doctors as powerful beings precisely because they have come to think of themselves as powerless prior to seeking treatment. But as any good doctor knows, great expectations can be dangerous, because if the patients go on to discover that their doctor is not God in sheep's clothing, they will feel betrayed, not just by the imperfect practitioner, but by the entire system. And even if the health professionals they have been dealing with maintain the very highest standards, they will still feel betrayed, simply because they will have been seeking guidance from a system that is there to serve the body first and the soul only if time and the budget allow.

But we are jumping ahead here; we are assuming that the patients have had access to all the new technologies medicine can offer. In fact, there is no such thing as fertility treatment on demand. First you have to prove yourself as the right kind of person. Requirements differ. Most have age limits, and almost all cost money. Some forms of treatment are closed to everyone except married couples. Even those that are open to single and lesbian women often insist on a psychiatrist's report. That is what happened to Alison and Cara when they approached a centre. 'We fought against it,' Alison recalls, 'but their reason was that they needed to cover their asses. People knew some specialists were inseminating lesbians. The psychiatrist turned out to be a good experience. I went once. She just told me she was there if we needed her, that she specialised in postnatal depression, and so on. It was fine. It took me two tries. The first time I miscarried and was very upset. But then the next time I got pregnant again and that time I carried her to term. I'd like to have another one eventually. Right now Cara is trying to get pregnant, but she's already on her fifth try. She's going to try one more time and then give up, because it's expensive. All straight people have to do is go out to the movies, but for us it's $450 a shot. We can't afford it.'

It is not only lesbian couples who have problems, talk to any single woman who tries to avail herself of fertility clinics, and you'll get a long catalogue of rejection and discrimination. 'Why didn't anybody tell me?' one such woman wailed. 'It's bad enough to have fertility problems, but on top of that, to keep hearing time and time again that according to these officious snots I'm not suitable . . .' If people really did make their family plans in the detached, measured and prudent way they make their housing, schooling, and even holiday plans, they would be keeping track of all these costs, requirements, and possibilities of discrimination. Unhappily, the usual thing is for people to assume they will be able to produce children at will – since clearly most people can – and only look into fertility treatments after at least a year of failing to do so. This puts them firmly into the category of the ailing patient with the defective body. Although pre-conceptual care is becoming more popular, there has been little movement in the direction of preconceptual awareness of possible fertility problems. By this we do not mean invasive tests or surgery are advisable, merely that people would be better off if they knew about the natural limits of fertility and the early indicators of fertility problems such as pelvic infections, endometriosis and, possibly, irregular periods.

Because this is so seldom the case, the norm is for the suffering, newly diagnosed patients to find themselves already too old for treatment, or unacceptable because of the wrong way of life, income level, or psychological profile. Vetting has a damaging effect even on the lucky people who qualify. The procedures may exacerbate their self-doubt and their feelings of being out of control. The longer it goes on – and remember, many couples will have to go on waiting lists after they have been accepted into a programme – the more their doubts and fears will grow. Although enlightened programmes may include counselling, reassurance, and support, there is still no substitute for the desperately wanted, non-appearing baby. This is the proof patients need before they can regain confidence in their fertility. From the point of view of the individual, in other words, it is not just fertility that is a means to an end. The baby, too, is a means to an end, because it is the baby who proves its parents' fertility. It's the baby that allows its parents to start thinking of themselves as important, productive, worthwhile people.

And if it doesn't appear?

'I always wanted to have a fourth child when I was thirty-eight,' says Eve, 'and of course I never did. I miss that child. I still think there's room for another young one around the house now. I do know everything about it. I'm sorry, but it's true. It's another little girl, and she's now about fourteen, and she goes to the — School, but she's more serious than my Selma. Oh dear, isn't that awful, I do know her very well, but Selma knows her well as well. She used to do pictures of her, saying, "That's me and my little sister what I do not have." Selma and I have invented her. But I do know her better than the three lost ones (from an abortion and two miscarriages) although I know them too. Frederick has an older brother who's rather serious, about twenty-six. . . . For those of us who've lost a baby, you don't know it, so it can sort of develop, you can put everything into it. It can be perfect.'

CHAPTER TEN

WHAT IS WRONG WITH THIS PICTURE?

It can be perfect. Or, as is the case for so many imaginary babies at the centre of so many fertility dilemmas, it can be the perfect monster who chews up futures between meals. Reproductive choices are, by definition, and for better or for worse, about imaginary babies. The language of choice is designed for the hypothetical. Even if an event has already occurred – for example a conception resulting in a child with Down's syndrome – the mother's decision to have an amniocentesis will be phrased in terms of risk. For the purposes of discussion, if not always for the pregnant woman, the baby isn't fully 'real' until it is born. To put it more strongly: fertility may be the ability to bear children, but feelings about fertility, and therefore fertility choices, often have little or nothing to do with children. Is this, we wonder, why people wrinkle their noses if a woman even suggests the possibility of putting a child she can't afford up for adoption? As one woman told us, 'When I said, just hypothetically, mind you, that I would rather give a child up for adoption than have an abortion, because of my religious beliefs, their response was, "Oh but how could you, how cruel could you get, you couldn't reject a child once you'd actually seen it, could you?" '

She concedes that she probably couldn't. And perhaps that's the crux of the problem. These are the rules of engagement. You can't make either/or decisions about other people's lives. You can only make them about your own. As one man said about the discussions he and his wife had before deciding to go ahead and have an unplanned child: 'It was a question of first things first. There wasn't a plan in place. We had to arrive at a position, and to do that we could not entertain the idea of the baby as a living thing. Because, you see, if we had thought of the baby as real, it would have been impossible even to phrase an either/or decision. There would have been no choice.'

In the past nine chapters, we have been looking at how people first come to the idea of having children, how they plan them, how they make use of contraception, how they handle surprises, what they go through when they're considering abortions or submitting themselves to genetic screening, how they come to decide on sterilisation, and how they are affected by unplanned fertility and fertility treatment.

Now let's stand back and look at the whole picture and see which patterns are suggesting themselves.

We're not quite sure why we want children in the first place. Try as we might to make our decisions to start a family sound rational, our original *wish* for a child is hard to justify in utilitarian terms. Broodiness seems to be a state of fairy-tale enchantment that descends on people out of the blue. Those of us who do not succeed in procreating immediately following the articulation of a wish for a child will often see the desire turn into an obsession – only to say afterwards, if we have had the good fortune of seeing the dream come true, that we cannot for the life us remember why we ever wanted children at all. (This rarely means that the children in question are not wanted: merely that the preconceived child bears little relation to the real one.)

Most of us pay some form of lip service to the ideals of family planning. In other words, we believe children should not arrive until we are 'ready'. A good nest is a must. Even though the rising divorce rate suggests that many planned children arriving into good nests will not be spending their entire childhoods there, still we cling to the idea that a baby deserves to be born in a nice, roomy house to a loving couple who enjoy a comfortable standard of living and are in a position to put home before work during the child's pre-school years. And yet, even those of us who meet the above standards will say afterwards that we had no idea what we were getting into (again, even if we are happy with the end results).

What Is Wrong With This Picture?

As for that other mainstay of the family ideal, the joint decision: as with Tolstoy's unhappy families, there are no two alike. While many married women still hold to the view that they are far better qualified to take charge of fertility matters, and that the ideal husband is the one who bows supportively to his wife's superior judgement, more and more men are expressing resentment at the degree to which they are left wringing their hands in the margins. Because there are no clear rules about what now passes for honourable conduct, each pair of prospective parents must come up with its own recipe – usually by trial and error. This often proves to be a dangerous game, because few people are able to say (or even know) in advance what principles are sacrosanct, what vows must never be bent during these negotiations. These usually only emerge after an irreversible betrayal.

Despite the high stakes, we continue to play roulette with contraceptives. While conscientious young women who have received ample sex education often report being happy and at ease with their chosen method, older women who have had to rely on contraception for a decade or two commonly express huge resentment, not just about the drawbacks of the various methods, but also about the day-to-day drudgery of contraceptive vigilance. As far as men are concerned, while some act like model citizens and never permit themselves unprotected sex unless they have made a conscious and carefully weighed decision to procreate, most have very patchy track records. If anything, the advances in the field of female contraceptives have reinforced the traditional idea that it is the woman who must make sure she does not conceive an inopportune child.

And if she does . . . the man will frequently assume that it has happened because the woman has planned it deliberately – and so will enter into the discussions on the fate of the pregnancy feeling just a little paranoid. This is one of the many reasons why these negotiations get off to a bad start. They are further complicated by the conviction that a woman is supposed to decide about an abortion on her own, and without anyone pressurising her. If you can imagine a man and a woman who believe no woman should be forced into either an abortion or an unwanted pregnancy, but who also believe that all children should result from a joint decision, you can see how quickly that couple is going to end up in a moral twilight zone.

As people in this twilight zone struggle to come to the 'right' decision, they will also be castigating themselves for their irresponsible, self-destructive contraceptive abuse, and further distressing themselves with the confusing discovery that they half want the ill-conceived child, and half don't want it. If they are feeling ambivalent now, they ask themselves, how are they going to feel if the baby ever sees the light of day? The baby grows to personify any number of threats and fears – and the bigger it gets, the less the real baby figures in the actual negotiations. Often women who discuss the prospect of abortion will go so far as to say afterwards that they don't believe they would have ever let themselves go ahead with it. Discussing abortion was for them a roundabout way of coming to accept the unexpected baby – a way of exercising a choice even though technically speaking they have already made that choice. The idea of abortion serves as a let-out clause.

And what form do the negotiations take? Decisions about abortions are almost always secret, but they are rarely made singly. The cast usually involves friends, partners, and family members as well as doctors. Their behaviour will have a bearing on the drama's resolution. That said, women who have had to face the big either/or question speak of feeling both 'totally in control' and 'desperately alone'. This is particularly true of women who have found themselves close to the cutting edge of reproductive technology.

Women who have had to make difficult fertility decisions often express their feelings by talking about their bodies – how reliable they are, how weak or powerful, who owns them, and how they have been treated by others. All this would suggest that fertility means an awful lot more than the ability to have children. It is also borne out by the words people use to describe their feelings about sterilisation. Many people who definitely don't want any or any more children dread the idea of losing the ability to procreate. It's almost as if fertility is the last remaining key to the afterlife. That said, many people who have been sterilised without being unduly pressurised speak of doing so to 'take control'.

What Is Wrong With This Picture?

The language of omnipotence flips over into the litany of defeat whenever people are confronted with unplanned infertility – in other words, whenever they find themselves unable to have sex, conceive children, or carry a pregnancy to term. Again, the obsession becomes the body, how it has failed, and what is being done to it. The non-appearing baby becomes idealised, and in some cases takes on a life of its own in the imagination of the would-be grieving parent. Men and women with imaginary children are loath to admit to them: if they do, they will couch their admission in apologies. But their children are no less imaginary than the children we desire when we first become broody, or the children whose fates we decide when contemplating an abortion, or mourn after a stillbirth or a miscarriage. The foundation on which the edifice of family planning sits is a fantasy.

That's why people can't explain the original desire to have children. That's why they plan so unrealistically and negotiate so haphazardly and make so many decisions they go on to resent or regret. That's why they play games with contraceptives – because feelings about fertility are not just utilitarian but symbolic and primitive and have far more to do with exercising power than they do with having children.

It would seem to follow, then, that if we are to manage our fertility better, we must confront and accept and tame, maybe even quell, these fantasies about bodies and babies. But saying that implies that there is something very dangerous about the power called fertility, and that vigilance is the only way to keep it in check.

We would beg to differ – and dare to suggest that many of the patterns we have described are not necessarily problems, or at least not problems that can be or need to be resolved. We *see* them as problems because the spectacles through which we are viewing them make them *look* like problems. In other words, it is our training that we ought to be examining as much as our behaviour. Because much of this derives from the medical understanding of fertility, our next stop will be the unhappy consultation room where we find ourselves obliged to implement so many of our hard-won choices.

CHAPTER ELEVEN

THE TROUBLE WITH DOCTORS

First, let's broaden the field. We're not just complaining about doctors, but also about nurses and counsellors and health educators – everyone, in fact, who delivers health care and health care information to the public.

What's wrong with them? They're biased – not all, thank God, in the same direction, but biased all the same. Most of us have strong ideas about other people's fertility. Doctors and other professionals are no exception. If they believe in the sanctity of life, they will honour that principle when advising candidates for abortion – sometimes subtly, sometimes not so subtly. If they believe that life on earth as we know it will end unless we control world population levels, they may not be entirely supportive of the uneducated teenager who wants to keep her baby, or the mother of five who has managed to get herself pregnant again just before she is due to go in to have her tubes tied. Like the rest of us, they have class and race prejudices. All too often, therefore, they apply one rule to the haves, and another to the have nots. The consultant who is cavalier about having to perform terminations on 'fifteen slags from Paddington' will say to a woman whom he sees as his social equal that 'our class of people don't do that kind of thing'. All too often, life in a married, middle-class womb is sacrosanct, and expendable wherever else it occurs. Abortion is a tragedy when it happens to 'us', a necessary form of birth control amongst the huddled masses of the developing world.

Although they are no better than the rest of us, health

professionals have set themselves as the moral arbiters of fertility. They judge us harshly if we reveal ourselves to have acted less than rationally. The result is two-tiered care. There is one rule for the sensible patient, and another for the patient who has been labelled 'self-destructive', 'chaotic', or 'undependable'. This means that any woman who wants to get the best treatment possible will take care to present herself as the former – even if this involves lying. She knows, for example, that her doctor is bound to think less of her or, at the very least, question her request for an abortion, if she admits that she deliberately chose not to use her diaphragm on the night of conception. Far easier, then, to say that the condom burst.

Here we begin to see that the present unhappy state of affairs is not entirely the fault of doctors. Who can blame them for persisting in judging patients by unrealistic standards if the patients themselves so often collude in this? If all patients were honest, health professionals would eventually have to change their standards. It is also true, however, that if all patients were honest, they would be complaining vociferously (as they did so often to us) about the way in which doctors pass on information.

When they prescribe contraceptives, for example, they don't say, 'Here's this packet of pills, here's how the pill works if you take your pill every day at the same time, and here's what happens if you miss your pill for two days running.' They say, 'Here's this packet of pills, and here's how you must take them.' They issue instructions, and so set up the expectation of obedience. Implicit is the idea that the patient cannot possibly have any legitimate motive *vis-à-vis* conception and contraception that the doctor has not foreseen. Patients who do not follow instructions are, as anyone who has ever looked at medical journals will know, classified as 'non-compliant'. If they get pregnant, the event is known as a 'contraceptive failure'.

It would be easier to take all this hand-wringing in medical journals about the problems created by irrational patients, if only the experts themselves were consistently rational. Alas, they fall way short. Primitive fairy-tale superstitions about the dangers of non-compliance lurk even in the terminology of birth control. There are Safe Days and Dangerous Days. People who exercise contraceptive 'vigilance' are 'protected'. People who have 'unprotected' intercourse run huge 'risks'. The implication is that you disobey the wizard's mysterious instructions at your peril. This message does not sit happily with the modern idea of the patient as someone who is supposed to be making her own decisions.

Which brings us to the problem of statistics. The recommended practice amongst good doctors today is to provide any woman facing a difficult fertility decision (fertility treatment, genetic screening, termination, sterilisation, and so on) with the most up-to-date information on the pertinent medical risks. A woman considering an amniocentesis will be told, for example, that the likelihood of someone her age carrying a Down's baby is 1 in 200, and the likelihood of the procedure itself causing a miscarriage 1 in 100. Likewise, a man considering a vasectomy will be told how likely it is that he could have a successful reversal, and how likely it is that he will have developed an antibody to his own sperm should he wait ten years before attempting a reversal. All this is to the good – and far better than the still common practice of giving patients too little information. What is not to the good is the expectation that it is possible to make a rational decision based on statistical odds.

It *is* possible to make a rational decision about public health policy based on statistical odds. For example, if twenty-five per cent of all women undergoing amniocentesis were to suffer miscarriages, it would be rational and practical for a hospital to decide that the risks involved in the procedure were too great for all but the two per cent of women who were most likely to be carrying Down's babies. But these figures are meaningless and impractical for the individual. Often the only sane response to such figures is an emotional one. But because this is not quite respectable, many people feel obliged to express their emotional decisions in intellectual terms. Consequently, they find themselves making emotional decisions without even realising that emotion was involved, without even being able to identify, let alone articulate their feelings.

What happens if patients do express their feelings? The common complaint is that they don't get respect for them. All too often doctors and nurses and hospitals act as if patients' feelings don't even exist. At best they treat their patients' feelings like mysterious ephemera that appear out of nowhere and do not go away unless handled like strange and growling dogs. All this serves to increase the already considerable mistrust patients feel towards their doctors. And it is very easy, if you feel you have been mistreated in any or all of the above-mentioned ways, to curse the day medicine decided to make fertility its business – and not too difficult to detect a nefarious conspiracy on the part of doctors to control women's bodies and therefore their destinies.

But before you jump, we would ask you to stop for a moment and remember how things were in the not-so-distant past.

Let's begin with sexual ignorance. Ask just about any woman over forty what kind of sex education she had, and she'll almost always be able to tell you an amusing story. We'll pass on a few here just to refresh your memory:

'After O level,' says Eve, 'we were given a talk at school as a reward. The speaker gave us an anatomically correct description of the sexual act, adding, "I am told it is pleasurable." My mother told me all about menstruation but nothing about conception because she was too embarrassed – even though she was a doctor.'

'I had one biology lesson in upper sixth, and the bare minimum from my mother,' recalls Eleanor. 'She gave me the facts of life one day while she was ironing.' Heather remembers: 'The textbook always said "like rabbits". The total concept of sex amongst adults was that it was like rabbits. Then we got someone from Marriage Guidance. There was an assumption you would have sex, and the talks were really about contraception, but not the nitty gritty, not "Here's a condom, here's a banana, get on with it," which seems to be the approach they take in schools today. It was all just talked about and very peculiar and there was an overall statement made about how you should really wait till you're married, and the rest was all geared to how not to get pregnant when you did it. We ended up with a weird combination of how you really shouldn't be doing this, i.e. guilt introduction, but if you're going to do it, don't get yourself pregnant. So you were left with a sort of weird feeling that sex was definitely guilt-ridden pre-marriage, but whatever you do, the important thing was to use contraception. The message was that if you had a baby it would wreck your career. . . .'

'I went to a parochial school,' remembers Frances. 'We got our instruction from a character we called Christ the Youth Leader. It was basic biological sex education. It began with slides. There would be a rabbit next to a lamppost, and then we were told that the difference between the rabbit and the lamppost was that the rabbit was alive and that it could reproduce. And it went on from there . . . how rabbits did it, how frogs did it and finally how humans did it, and yes, there was the moment of climax, which we had beautifully described for us. We used to recite it to each other when we went out for walks: "He kisses her, he cuddles her, he tells her that he wants her, then he thrusts his engorged penis into her. . . ." She used to blush very easily, this woman. After that, Catholic Marriage Guidance came along and talked about how to say no, and how to conduct contraception through the rhythm method, and how there was always abstention. . . .' A well-known health educationalist recounts her own early sex education at school: it was to knit a uterus!

When women over forty go on to describe their early sexual experiences, almost every problem they run into comes from catastrophic innocence. 'I thought I couldn't get pregnant if we did it standing up.' 'He told me he was using protection and so not to worry. I had no idea what he meant or what protection looked like and so I simply trusted him.' 'How was I meant to know instinctively that this man I was about to marry was homosexual? I never even heard the word homosexual until I was thirty!' Single women who had the courage to seek contraceptive advice before the 1967 Family Planning Act speak also of public humiliation. 'In her loudest voice, in front of a full waiting room, the lady behind the desk said, "We don't do that kind of thing for unmarried women!" '

And next time you're fretting over the problems presented by legalised abortion, remember these stories about illegal abortion. Blanche, a single ballet dancer without a family who found herself pregnant after a brief fling with someone for whom she had little admiration or affection, gave herself a saline abortion. It took several days to work, she recalls. One of her roommates was a medical student and did what he could to help her through it. 'We turned it into a joke. I remember us all laughing about how the fetus looked like Horatio, the father.' They got rid of it by flushing it down the loo. 'People told me I would feel terrible afterwards, but in fact I felt nothing.' Hazel, who suffered a severe abdominal infection after a back-street abortion when she was a nineteen-year-old student, has never been able to conceive a child since. Andrea, who was a missionary when she found herself pregnant, like Blanche and Hazel would have faced destitution and disgrace had she chosen to continue with it. Despite ever more desperate attempts, she was five months gone before she found anyone willing to abort it. As they threw it casually into the sink, they told her it was a boy and asked her if she wanted to take a look. Because she believed it was wrong to rope a man into marriage with a pregnancy, and because she wasn't sure of her own affections for him, she didn't tell the father until afterwards, although, she says, he must have guessed because of her distress. His response was, 'Oh darling, you're so brave.' She believes that the reason they got married soon afterwards was out of respect for their lost child.

And let's finish off with a midwife remembering the day she told her mother (born at about the turn of the century) about her decision to go into this field of medicine. ' "Oh, you don't want to do that," my mum said. "You don't want to be a midwife. You'll have to smother all the defective ones." I said, "What?" And she said that was what midwives had to do in her day, to gently smother the defective ones at birth. That was the way it was, she said, when most women had their babies at home.'

There are plenty of people arguing today for a return to traditional values, but few would willingly return themselves, or anyone they knew and loved, to vulnerable ignorance, unsafe medical procedures, and public humiliation. And while many of us are wary of the implications of fertility having gone public, and are anxious to retain control over our bodies and our reproductive rights, we can still see that doctors are not the evil genies that we sometimes suspect them to be. Life after medical choice is definitely a better place than life when fertility was private and 'natural'. The project, then, is not to turn the clock back, but to learn better how to read it.

CHAPTER TWELVE

A BEAUTIFUL PICTURE

Meet Frances. She is twenty-nine years old and has just begun as the junior partner of an established but forward-looking general practice. What understanding of fertility does she bring with her to her first day of work?

She will be well acquainted with the physiological processes of reproduction – and will respect them for their efficiency, fragility and subtle harmonies. She will see her job as either impeding these processes, or helping them along their way, depending on her individual patient's aims and needs. Although the terminology she must use will tend to the mechanical, she will, because of her extensive knowledge of natural family planning, be hoping to promote fertility awareness – in other words encouraging patients to get to know how their own bodies work – instead of just comparing themselves to scientific norm.

She is against the old authoritarian mode that was once the norm amongst general practitioners. She believes that her job is to provide patients with the wherewithal to make their own informed choices. She is determined never to impose her own solutions on patients, especially when they are making life or death decisions. While it will be her responsibility to provide the time and space and information the patient needs before making such decisions, Frances has already made a resolve to respect the patient's wishes even when she cannot understand or condone them. If a teenager wants an IUD put in despite data suggesting that it is not the safest method for a young and childless woman; if a man asks for a vasectomy but does not wish to inform his wife; if a woman who wants to start a family at twenty-eight requests a termination when she becomes accidentally pregnant at twenty-seven, it will be Frances' duty, after due consideration, to provide them with the devices and services they request so long as they are permitted under the law. She is also planning to do her best to make all the information she gives as 'patient-friendly' as possible.

Because she is an exceptionally thoughtful person, she will have given long consideration to the consequences of reproductive choice. Common sense has already told her that it is easier to accept an accident than it is to initiate a plan, especially for a woman who cannot expect her partner to support her while she brings up their children. She plans to bear these facts of modern life in mind when she counsels couples. She also plans to bear in mind the fact that the new reproductive technologies have created new problems for the patient by blurring the boundaries of the possible. In fact, she has just read a very good article about the new pressures on infertile couples now that it is no longer easy to adopt. As she parks her car in the designated space, she recalls its wise words: 'Whereas childless people in the past sometimes needed counselling to come to terms with their childlessness, the current situation is more complex. There are choices to be explored, outcomes to be weighed carefully, hidden agendas to be brought out into the open, and complex medical technology to be understood.'[1]

Yes, thinks Frances as she double-checks the locks on her car. The guide through the jungle of statistics, the wise enabler – this is what she wants to be, she tells herself as she sits down at her new desk. It's nine a.m. The surgery has started. She presses the buzzer to admit her first patient.

Imagine how perplexed she will be by the end of the first day if the people in the waiting room have anything in common with the people we have quoted in previous chapters.

Some will have lied to her – out of fear and embarrassment – but still, it doesn't make her job any easier. Some will practically demand that she makes up their minds for them. Some will come in on Monday expressing a wish for one service, and on Wednesday requesting the opposite. Others will seem unable to take on board the simplest set of instructions. Few people will give any indication that they want to understand – let alone respect – their bodies. Only rarely will she meet up with a patient who seems sure of his or her own mind, who is comfortable weighing medical risk factors, and who seems likely to follow all instructions responsibly. But many of these apparently reliable patients will also prove disquieting. Is it possible to be sure, for example, that a thirty-one-year-old woman who definitely does not ever want to have children will feel exactly the same way in her late thirties? It is one thing to make a blanket advance resolution about respecting other people's decisions. It is another to sit in a room with a patient whose certainty looks very much like a very thin sheet of ice covering a very deep pool of unexamined feelings.

Frances is not the only one to be perplexed. Speak to any sensitive, enlightened counsellor or doctor, and you'll soon discover that it is not just the professionals who cling to the old ways. Just as some doctors tend to be paternalistic, so do many patients want doctors to issue edicts. And when doctors refuse to do so, the patients are confused and angry and complain that the doctor is not doing his or her job. One doctor we spoke to gave us the example of a patient who found out she was pregnant not long after her husband went into prison. When the authorities told her to have an abortion, it was easy for her rebel and have the baby. But when she sought counselling from her new doctor about a second pregnancy, and was told that it was her life, and her decision, she was terribly distressed and didn't know what to do. 'When a woman is not accustomed, or not willing to make her own decisions, the counsellor's job becomes almost impossible. Successful counselling requires a partnership, and I'm afraid that when you can't establish it, the only recourse is to be directive. I try very hard to make clients realise that we're here to work with them, and that the choices are theirs, that they don't have to tell a particular story or fit a particular profile in order to qualify for an abortion. I know it falls very short of the ideal to be directive when that is the framework, but there are times when I know that if I don't do it, this woman will go and ask the person standing next to her at the bus stop. It's not something I like to do. It's a last resort.'

The lost ideal behind this and so many other legitimate complaints is the patient as informed decision-maker. The experienced doctor, counsellor, nurse and health educator will have learned over and over again that few human beings match up to it. When they ask themselves why, the answer is usually ignorance, and the solution therefore better education and more accessible, consumer-centred information. Where this proves to be not enough, then the verdict becomes 'chaotic' or 'self-destructive behaviour'. And if a patient is self-destructive, doesn't it follow that a responsible health professional might be obliged to take steps on occasion to 'save the patient from herself'?

But what if part of the problem is the doctor's expectation of the patient – if the model of the patient as rational decision-maker is faulty?

In the feminist classic, *Thinking About Women*, Mary Ellmann describes beautifully the discrepancy between a woman's understanding of her body and the way right-thinking family planners see it:

'Women must be partially conscious, in witnessing any disorder (however apparently purposeful or deliberate), of emerging from disorder as well. Their physiology is not one from which confidence in executive procedure can be extracted. Menstruation proves that the body carries out expensive, time-consuming and futile operations. The retraction of the uterine wall, which leaves the inflated veins to atrophy, break open and lose their absurd provisions for a non-event, constitutes an image of repeated bankruptcy. A monthly reminder that failure is as likely as success, and that failure may sometimes be as welcome as success – principles which, obviously, do not govern our society. . . . At the same time, women cannot help observing that conception (their highest virtue, by all reports) simply happens or doesn't. It can be prevented by foresight and device . . . but it is accomplished by luck (good or bad). Purpose often seems, if anything, a deterrent. A devious business, benefiting from indirection, by pretending not to care, as though the self must trick the body. In the regrettable conception, the body tricks the self

– much as it does in illness or death. It is probably in consequence of this physical sense of double-dealing that women do not – at any rate convincingly – endorse evangelical views of sexual intercourse. Sober self-congratulation is impeded for them by the ever-present possibility of becoming the butt of a joke. Nor can women think properly in terms of the conservation or frugal distribution of sexual materials. The easy fusion, for men, of a capitalistic and physical ethic must bemuse women, whose chief sexual (if not spiritual) characteristic is an ungovernable extravagance. In fact, to any entrepreneur except nature, the human female would seem too wasteful to keep in stock.'[2]

Experienced health professionals are aware that fertility means more to their patients than just the ability to have children. They call these extraneous agendas 'emotional', with the implication that they are irrational, and even where they make allowances for them, they have a hard time justifying them. If you have a utilitarian understanding of fertility, they make no sense.

We believe that if they had a broader definition of fertility, and a less mechanistic understanding of how people make their decisions, these extraneous agendas would not just make sense but underpin their every consultation.

We would like to suggest an alternative model of the patient: instead of an informed decision-maker, a calculated risk-taker.

We take our inspiration from Kristin Luker, author of *Taking Chances*, a groundbreaking and still influential study of selected Californian abortion clinics in the early seventies. In it she points out that the official attitude inside the health establishment and the family planning movement 'is that any pregnancy which is unwanted should have been prevented, or at least should have a history of attempts at prevention. If no attempts were made to prevent it, then the female (rarely does this analysis extend to the male half of the couple) is at best irrational and at worst pathological.' She goes on to point out that women define the situation differently. 'In making decisions about contraception they try to attain many goals, only one of which is not getting pregnant.' It is only after becoming pregnant 'that women face the prevailing definition of the situation

– that any pregnancy which was not actively prevented is irrational and inexplicable – and thus begin to feel they must be either irrational or confused about what they really want.'[3]

Sex is a private event. So is the decision to use or forgo contraception. Pregnancy, on the other hand, is a condition of social significance. It involves a large cast of mothers, fathers, sisters, brothers, partners, and health professionals who may not have the final say about whether the pregnancy goes forward or not, but whose opinions have weight, and whose disapproval can cause great distress – as well as practical difficulties. It is perfectly possible, and normal, for a teenage girl to decide, in the safety and privacy of her own room, that she wants to have a baby, only to find that her decision looks foolish in the cold light of a positive pregnancy test. If the father denies responsibility, if her parents tell her a baby at this stage will wreck her life, she may become frightened and change her mind. If other people think of her behaviour as irrational, she will, if she is of an impressionable age, be tempted to deny her original motives and pass the same judgement on herself – regardless of whether or not she goes ahead with the pregnancy. The same pattern can occur in older and married women, especially in marriages where children are meant to arrive as a result of a joint decision – even when the matter of contraception is left entirely to the wife. A woman who has conceived because of a unilateral decision not to use contraception, or because she assumed there was a tacit agreement to have a child, may be similarly tempted to reclassify her behaviour as irresponsible if her partner responds negatively to the news that she is pregnant. A privately wanted child can quickly become a public mistake. In other words, many people take contraceptive risks because, at the time, they find the possibility of pregnancy an attractive one. If they change their minds afterwards, it is because their own feelings are complicated by the evidence of domestic outrage, or because the social costs are far higher than they imagined.

This is not to say that all women seeking abortions do so because of social pressure, or that all people who take contraceptive risks want babies. There is such a thing as an unwanted pregnancy. Why does it happen? The traditional view – and the assumption upon which the family planning movements both here and in the US were founded – is contraceptive ignorance. Today's family planning experts take this theory with a grain of salt – it is generally agreed that information alone is not enough to get people to use contraception 'responsibly'. Also discredited is another once very popular explanation, the 'intra-psychic conflict theory', which sees women as possessing the necessary contraceptive skills but experiencing resistance against using them. Although it is still commonplace for discussions of contraceptive failure in medical journals and in the mass media to see the 'problem' as belonging to the woman, many family planning professionals believe, like Kristin Luker, that the theory is methodologically weak, does not account for social changes, ignores the social and demographic aspects of contraceptive behaviour, and is misogynist.[4]

Her own still controversial theory is that unwanted pregnancy results from 'contraceptive risk-taking behaviour which is the result of conscious decision-making'.[5] Every time a woman has to make a decision about contraception (if she is using a barrier method this will mean every time she has intercourse; if she is on the pill this will mean every time she is due to take a tablet) she weighs the 'disadvantages and benefits of contraception against the disadvantages and benefits of an unwanted pregnancy'.[6] Often the 'immediate costs of contraception' will appear greater than the 'anticipated benefits of pregnancy'.[7] If she does not want to define herself as a sexually active woman, if she thinks contraception kills spontaneity, if she is going to have to wait another three weeks before her appointment at the clinic, if she is underage and can't afford contraception, if she has stopped using the pill after breaking up with her partner and then finds herself unexpectedly reunited with him, or if she finds her chosen method upsetting or inconvenient, she may be inclined to take a chance. She will be even more inclined if she thinks she is unlikely to become pregnant. Pregnancy is 'a probability of known magnitude'[8] for statisticians. If a hundred sexually active women of childbearing age go without contraception for a year, eighty of them will become pregnant – but for an individual it is an uncertainty. ('You can't become eighty per cent pregnant.')[9] If she thinks of herself, or has been categorised by a doctor, as sub- or infertile, contraceptive vigilance may not seem to be worth the trouble or expense.[10] She may also have positive feelings about pregnancy. To be pregnant is to prove that she is fertile, and a 'real woman'. It is to challenge and perhaps redefine her relationship with her family and her partner, force a commitment, demand status.[11] 'We believe that all sexually active women are potential risk-takers,' says Kristin Luker. '. . . Safe, cheap abortion lowers the ante.'[12]

Warren B. Miller, who has taken on board Luker's ideas without fully rejecting the idea that a woman can act against her own best interests, has found that women are particularly 'vulnerable to unwanted pregnancy' at times of transition − during early adolescence, when she may still be sub-fecund or sterile and has not redefined herself as a sexual being; when she first becomes sexually active, and has not had time to seek contraceptive advice; when she is just entering a stable relationship, before the 'necessary contraceptive negotiations' have been carried out; when that stable relationship is in crisis, and normal patterns of co-operation and responsible behaviour break down; when she moves to a new place with different mores, for example, university; when she is about to get married; when she has just had a child or an abortion; when she is approaching the end of her childbearing period; and when she is coming up to menopause.[13] In every instance, her contraceptive behaviour will be the result of a complex and largely intuitive sifting process. She will be weighing up the (perceived) pros and cons of pregnancy against the (perceived) costs and benefits of contraception. She will be taking into account what her partner thinks and does, and also be influenced by friends, family, the media, and also by the attitudes of the people who actually provide the contraceptives in her community. Also important are her feelings and ideas about contraception in general and her chosen method in particular. Some methods require more will-power than others. If a woman hasn't had all the children she wants to have, and she is using a barrier method, she will tend to become 'relaxed' about contraception. The same thing happens where motivation is 'subconscious'. Miller sees subconscious motivation as conforming to three different types of thoughts: '(1) At times I have a half-wish to get pregnant or have a baby, although I know it's not practical, (2) there are times when I just don't care whether or not I get pregnant, and (3) I am the sort of woman who might get pregnant just to hurt or punish myself. . . . Thus, when a woman cannot completely suppress her wish to become pregnant in spite of important situational constraints, when a woman loses the psychological energy that is continuously required to avoid conception, or when a woman feels the urge to use becoming pregnant as a way of dealing with certain negative feelings about herself, then her contraceptive practice tends to become inconsistent and ineffective.'[14] (Again, note the value judgement: according to Warren B. Miller, relaxed contraceptive use is always a kind of failure.)

He found different patterns of contraceptive use amongst married and unmarried women. The former did better with contraceptives if they stayed away from barrier methods and used the pill or the IUD, if they were emotionally stable, and if they had higher levels of education. The latter did better if they had fewer partners and more frequent intercourse.[15]

He based these findings on the Psychology of Reproduction Study, an extensive four-year study begun in the San Francisco Bay area in 1972. Its thousand subjects were divided into three groups: women who had never married, women who had just married and were childless at the outset, and women who had just given birth to their first child. It is not clear to us why older women were not made part of the study – is it assumed that married mothers have contraception all figured out? We are also mystified – and so are many professionals writing in the field – as to why this and so many other studies of abortion and contraceptive behaviour focus solely on women. As Mary Boyle says, 'an alien reading some of the research [on this subject] would have to conclude that men had nothing to do with either contraception or conception.'[16] One reason for the bias is, she thinks, the fact that women provide a 'captive subject-pool for family planning clinics, pregnancy advisory services, termination clinics, and mother and baby homes'.[17] Because society sees fertility as women's business, research reflects this assumption, too. She feels this 'selective attitude' to women 'places an unfair burden on them and makes it more difficult for men to share the responsibility for contraception even if they wished to do so.'[18]

In other words, people often take risks because they don't know what the rules are. As Kristin Luker notes, 'recent changes in the technology of contraception and in the ideology of the sexual revolution have left some people at a loss as to who has what obligations in a sexual relationship. When people have a tenuous relationship, or when they fear the feeling of "couplehood" that joint decision-making implies, there appears to be a tendency for both of them to postpone action because each expects the other to take the dominant role.'[19]

There is clearly some truth in this, but there is also something missing in this as well as the other analyses we have considered in this chapter. Perhaps they are asking the wrong question. Perhaps it should be – considering how complicated and difficult and riddled with uncertainties everyday life is for most people – why is it that people don't take risks more often?

We would like to suggest that we all do, all day long.

Just as we take calculated risks every time we venture out on a motorway – weighing the probable costs of an accident against the benefits to be gained by, for example, changing lanes – just as we take calculated risks every time we eat, drink, or even venture into our own kitchen, so we take risks every time we have intercourse. After all, no form of contraception is one hundred per cent effective. It is also important to remember that our primary aim when we have intercourse is rarely, and maybe even never, to test out the effectiveness of our chosen contraceptive. We have other aims in mind – lots of them. We may have plenty of reasons to fear pregnancy, but as we lie there on that bed or beach or floor or car seat, we may also have plenty of reasons to welcome the idea. Every time we have sex, we'll be intuitively sifting through all these wishes and fears. Every time we have sex, they will balance out differently

A Beautiful Picture

and so possibly lead to a different level of risk-taking. For example, a woman who wants a second child in about two years' time, who knows that her cycle is usually thirty-one days, and who has sex without contraceptives a week before she usually ovulates, is taking a risk she will have little trouble living with. A man who would like a child, but who is afraid that if he brings up the idea, his partner will say that she will only agree to it so long as he gives up his job to care for the child full-time, will, it could be said, be taking a risk that is very much to his tactical advantage if he pretends not to notice that his partner has become lax about contraception. When medical experts talk about risks, they are usually alluding to possible negative outcomes of a particular course of action. What we would like to suggest is that the kind of everyday risk-taking we engage in – both on and off the bed – is usually a hopeful exercise, and often a fruitful one. Nothing ventured, nothing gained, after all. Taking a risk in an uncertain world is a way of taking a calculated, and limited, degree of control.

Everyday intuitive risk-taking is specific and usually happens so quickly it looks and feels automatic. It is only when you look back at a particular risk you took that you have time to philosophise. Making an informed choice is, by contrast, a hugely symbolic and self-conscious exercise. You are convinced, or made to feel as if you are standing at one of the great cross-roads of life. You have been living consistently according to one rational game-plan: now you are considering a new, revised game-plan. Which offers the best deal? It is easy, when you are thinking this way, to imagine that you have more control over your future than anyone on earth actually does. It is also easy, both before and after you have made the 'big decision', to idealise, elaborate and torture yourself with visions of the path not taken. The threat of regret plays a far larger part in our deliberations than most of us would care to admit. 'If you have an abortion, it will haunt you forever.' 'If you have a child too young, it will wreck your life.' 'Single women who get pregnant don't know what they're letting themselves in for.' Anyone who has faced a difficult fertility decision will remember being haunted, and confused, by such remembered admonitions. The implication is that any choice that leads to regret is a mistake.

What we would like to suggest is that all choices involve loss and regret, and that the path not taken is always the plaything of the imagination. It can become the cautionary tale ('Just imagine how horrible my life would be now if I had had that child/that abortion . . .') or, if the path taken becomes too unpleasant, the untried alternative can be shaped into perfection – shaped and enjoyed. It is always impressive to see the loving detail with which people can describe the travels and careers and fat bank accounts they went without for the sake of children, and even more moving, the imaginary children some women invent after a miscarriage or an abortion. These are hypothetical lives – useful fantasies, but not to be confused with the life history without which these choices have no meaning.

When we talk about difficult choices we have made, we describe strong and mysterious emotions suddenly springing up out of nowhere. Because they are as surprising as they are difficult to control, and because they are not *meant* to get in the way when we're making a rational decision, we describe them as irrational, silly, totally insane, and try to push them aside. But disowning such emotions makes them even stronger and much harder to control, and a wiser course is to entertain the possibility that they might have a home.

When we approach an important fertility decision, we spend a lot of time trying to guess how we might feel in the future. This straining for prescience makes it hard to bear in mind – and later to remember – the exact context in which we are making the decision, i.e. what we know at that precise moment in time, and what we are not to know. When we take risks, however, or when we see our past decisions as exercises in risk-taking, we usually have a very clear idea of the context in which we took those risks, as well as a shrewd assessment of the degree of uncertainty involved. A risk is a jump into the unknown. There is, from the very beginning, an acknowledgement that there may be a certain amount of loss. If the timing of the risk, and its reason, and its nature are based on a 'gut feeling', this is not the same as saying it is reckless or based on fickle emotions. A 'gut feeling' is more likely to be shorthand for that

A Beautiful Picture

complex, intuitive sifting that Kristin Luker and Warren B. Miller mention.

The obsessive and self-castigating regretter is the person who has forgotten where she was standing at the moment when she had to make her decision, what the world looked like, what she wanted at that point in time, what she feared, what she knew and what she could never have predicted. If she were able to step back into the shoes she was wearing at the time, she would probably still wish she had acted differently, but she would have a harder time calling the decision a mistake. And, if she thought about it for a while, she would probably also realise that every agonising conscious choice she made was preceded and succeeded by hundreds of little decisions she made without even realising, thousands of calculated risks she took on the basis of automatic, 'instinctive' judgements, the kind of quick but complicated judgements we make when we're merging with traffic on a motorway or walking down a crowded pavement. It is the sum total of all these moment-in-time decisions, big and small, conscious and automatic, that gives us our life story. And why do we find our life story so surprising? Because so many of our decisions are guided by the emotional preferences we tend to leave out of our big, sensible, rational 'plans for life'. 'I always thought I would have children,' says one woman, 'but I guess in the end I didn't want them enough. This surprises me. I had no idea my work was that important to me.' Another woman says what seems to be the opposite: 'I was and still am extremely ambitious, so I can't figure out (a) why I've ended up with so many children and (b) why it makes me so happy. I can only conclude that I must like children.' What both women had in common, though, was an ambivalence about having children. They were 'in two minds', and only time, and a chain of big and little decisions, would reveal which 'mind' would win out.

'For ten years – from the time I was twenty-eight to the time I was thirty-eight – I was totally obsessed with getting pregnant. Eventually I was lucky enough to have two children, thanks to IVF. But now that I have them, to tell you the truth, I can't remember why I ever wanted them. I don't know if I even *like* children.'

'My children are the most important part of my life, but if it had been left to me, I wouldn't have had any. It was my wife who made the decisions and imposed them on me.'

'The one thing I knew for sure was that I couldn't abide having a Down's child. The only reason I didn't have an amnio was that they told me it was highly unlikely for a woman in my age bracket. But now here I am with a Down's child, and he's the best thing that ever happened to me.'

'I'm very sorry now that I got what I wanted when I was twenty-one. Life would have been a hell of a lot easier if I hadn't had two small children in tow.'

What are these people saying with their stories of regret and reprieves? Simply that they feel differently about a particular plan or wish or decision now than they did at the time when they still had a choice. If this change of outlook makes them say they made a mistake, this is partly due to the language of family planning and the expectations to which this language gives rise. We would like to suggest that no family planning strategy is foolproof, precisely because such changes of heart are always possible.

We would even go farther and suggest that even the most prudent family planning strategy involves risk. If you take the pill for fifteen years, you risk not being able to conceive on demand. If you have a baby at fifteen, you risk missing out on schooling and a carefree adolescence. If you conceive a child at the most auspicious time, you still run a risk of having a miscarriage. There is no such thing as perfect knowledge: while we will be aware of some of the risks we are taking in following a particular course, we will never know all of them. So why do we blame ourselves when things don't work out perfectly? Because we talk about 'family planning' rather than 'family risking'. The motto of Planned Parenthood of America is: 'Children by choice, not chance'. What is the unintended message behind this laudable aim? We would say it is an invitation to harsh self-judgement. A risk is something you take because you can't achieve x without running a y per cent chance of negative outcome z. If you get negative outcome z, you are unlucky, but if you have implemented a plan that hasn't worked out, you have failed.

A Beautiful Picture

And if you have gone into the original planning with an exaggerated idea of the degree to which your future is under your control, you are all the more likely to exaggerate your personal responsibility for any failure. All too often, agreeing to hold the hot potato becomes taking blame for the hot potato – much of which can belong with other people. As we have pointed out in earlier chapters, even the most personal decisions are made within severe social constraints. Often it is not the baby that causes the problem, but the ordeal of fitting the baby in with the rest of one's life – as institutions are set up for the family with one stay-at-home parent and another parent with an income that is twice the national average.

The official term for such glaring injustices is 'social constraints'. They are much easier to identify in a specific instance of risk-taking than they are in a large, symbolic decision, because the latter is so often based on an inflated idea of the degree to which we are able to shape our future.

If we worked from the model of human being as calculated risk-taker, rather than expecting ourselves to be corporate decision-makers who never have occasion to look back; if we understood ourselves to be playing a complex juggling game every time we took a risk, and agreed that no result is ever 'right' enough to make the risk-taker immune to regret, we would waste less time trying to 'make sense' of our behaviour and more time handicapping the risks we need to take. What's more, by examining the risks we have already taken, we can get a clearer idea of what we really want, or where we are ambivalent, or which of two opposite inclinations is stronger.

And if health professionals worked from this model, it would quickly become clear that 'how to' instructions are not enough when it comes to contraception. Having acknowledged that a normal human being will often have as many good reasons not to use contraception as reasons to use it, the information would be redesigned so that the patient is clear not just about how the device works if she follows the instruction, but what will happen if she uses it sporadically or stops altogether.

If getting pregnant without overt premeditation were no longer thought to be the result of self-destructive behaviour until proven otherwise, counselling patients about what to do about these pregnancies would get off to a far better start.

And if sex education were based on the idea that fertility is a power you can manage through intelligent risk-taking, instead of a dark force to be repressed through relentless social conditioning, students would be able to draw upon their sex education through life. Today, the chief aim of sex education is to prevent teenage pregnancy. Its lessons can be extremely counterproductive when people apply them in later life. All too often 'fertility control' can mean 'fertility obedience'. This scenario sets up the possibility for its opposite, fertility disobedience – whereas if you are taking and managing and assessing your own risks, you can't be disobedient, because in a sense you are your own boss.

What we are trying to say, then, is that we could solve many big problems just by correctly interpreting our behaviour, and basing our strategies on a more realistic model of the model patient. But even if all involved saw the light tomorrow, and altered their lives accordingly, even if all the doctors and nurses and planners and educators in the world became less directive, and all the patients in the world more assertive, there would still be other serious problems that no amount of democratic negotiation, no amount of healthy soul-searching could ever resolve. The new birth technologies continue to create moral dilemmas where none existed before. These are not just the obvious ones you read about in the paper – the breakthroughs in gender selection techniques, and surrogacy, and post-menopausal pregnancy – but also the less publicised contradictions that exist inside most of our hospitals. One of the more disturbing instances of this – and one which we will be examining in greater detail later – is the way in which advances in neonatology and fertility treatments have crossed wires with advances in genetic screening – so making a mockery of the current legal limits on abortion. At present, abortion is legal up to twenty-four weeks – and yet babies born as early as twenty-two or twenty-three weeks are being routinely saved. It is hard to reconcile the fact that on one floor of a hospital they will be trying to save babies born at twenty-three

A Beautiful Picture

weeks, while on a different floor they are throwing babies, and probably healthier babies, of the same gestation, into the incinerator. The fact that it happens puts a great strain on all people working close to the actual patients. The unsolved moral dilemma trickles down to them. The only thing they can do if they stay in the job is put on blinkers. As one counsellor who works with late terminations commented, 'You have to cope with it, because you have to say, "I am looking after this person, the person who has made this decision, and this person deserves to be looked after in the most efficient medical manner that I am capable of doing, to set her off to start again." That's the way I cope with it. Everybody has to be looked at as an individual. You can't link the whole of the hospital together.'

A second area of moral difficulty has to do with certain methods of family planning. Some of the new devices at times allow fertilisation of the egg, but disrupt implantation. There is consequently a drive to downplay the importance of fertilisation and to say that life does not begin until a fertilised egg has implanted. A third area of difficulty is the new abortion pill, which could make abortion much more like the personal private choice we already pretend it to be, but which could also provide a convenient way for doctors and other pillars of society to continue doing what they already do too much – which is to pretend that problem pregnancies are the woman's responsibility and the woman's fault. The new reproductive technologies are bringing us closer and closer to the time when parents will be able to custom order their offspring. At the same time, health services and insurance companies will soon be able to withhold treatment and coverage from those babies whose parents allow them to see the light of day despite genetic screening that has revealed undesirable or costly defects. While the debate drags on as to where we ought to draw the legal lines, patients and doctors must resolve these moral dilemmas on a case-by-case basis and must live with the guilt and stress that the contradictions of birth technology have produced.

In such conditions, the enlightened health professional's admirable efforts to make sure patients make their own decisions begin to look more like passing the hot potato. If you can convince yourself that you're there to serve the patient's wishes, then you can avoid the full brunt of a moral decision. The words 'wanted' and 'unwanted', 'planned' and 'unplanned' provide the means by which health professionals can avoid taking responsibility for what they find themselves forced to do. To examine these terms becomes a highly dangerous exercise – if you are convinced that the buck stops with the doctor.

In fact, fertility is not just my business and your business and the doctor's business, but – for better or for worse – *everybody's* business.

CHAPTER THIRTEEN

FERTILITY IS POLITICAL

Since when? I hear you ask. Alas, from the beginning of time, because whoever controls it sets the agenda for the next generation. We all have glorious dreams about the 'better world' our children and grandchildren could inhabit, if only today's world agreed to regulate procreation according to our recommendations. It is not just human to be political about fertility. It is humanitarian – though not, as we shall see, particularly humane.

But first let's meet the four classic fertility utopians who are dominating the debate today.

We'll begin with Doctor Dreamer. He can trace a huge number of the social problems that plague us back to illness, ignorance, bad health habits, and families that are too large for existing resources. In his ideal world, the society of healthy, well-informed, socially responsible adults manage their reproductive systems in a respectful way, while the medical establishment works with them to help them beget the perfect number of auspiciously timed, healthy, normal children.

Seemingly at odds with Doctor Dreamer is Petronella Pro-Life. Although she has great sympathy for single women who choose parenthood over abortion and will work hard to support them in that effort, she sees many modern evils as having emanated from the destruction of the traditional family. In her utopia, all babies are alive and universally accepted as such from the moment of conception – and born into traditional families headed by male breadwinners and supervised by nurturing stay-at-home mothers.

At the third side of our negotiating table sits Peggy Pro-Choice. She sees our main problem today as coming from the continuing efforts on the part of the male establishment to oppress the other half of humanity. In her ideal world, each individual woman is making her own reproductive choices and only has the children she can afford to fit into her life-plan. These children may or may not have active fathers.

The fourth utopian at the table is Fred Family Planner, who sees many of the world's worst problems as coming from the wrong people having too many children for the wrong reasons at the wrong time. His programme is to eradicate overpopulation by promoting the idea of the small family both here and in the developing world, and to limit crime, poverty, endemic drug-use, and child abuse by bringing down the pregnancy rate amongst teenagers and other high-risk groups. His ideal world, in other words, is a place where people make their own choices – but would never dream of a choice that wasn't socially responsible.

What do all four idealists have in common? They all want to use the same vehicle to arrive at their respective utopias. The fertile woman is the key. Whoever controls her heart and mind, determines the future of humanity.

Another thing they all share is a shaky foundation in history. This is not surprising, as it is not in their interest to improve it. Their aim is not to understand the links between the present and the past but to win followers. And so they base their campaign speeches on commonly accepted generalisations that have little truth in them, because the truth, as usual, is a bit too complicated. The traditional family was never quite the solid institution people think it was. Women were never quite the abject baby machines feminists think they were. There is no clear conspiracy of patriarchs. Doctors have frequently been at odds with fathers, and family planning is not a modern phenomenon.

We can find an interest in birth control going back to the beginning of history. The Egyptians had contraceptive paste; the Greeks had douches and may have invented the IUD; the Talmud permitted Jewish women to use tampons and an oral contraceptive

Fertility is Political

containing pounded crocuses. Moslem women used potions and pessaries. In medieval Europe, midwives dispensed their own herbal remedies. The condom and the Dutch cap have been with us for centuries. Throughout the ages, prolonged breast-feeding has limited family size.[1] Overlaying, or infanticide, has also long been suspected to be a popular last-resort measure. And in the West in particular, there has been the time-honoured tradition of late marriage.

When we castigate ourselves for our half-baked modern families, we often do so by harking back to the Traditional Family, to the good old days when women had no careers and so married young and had lots and lots of children as a matter of course. In fact, demographic family historians have been able to establish that during the seventeenth, eighteenth and nineteenth centuries, the average first marriage age in Western Europe was twenty-seven or twenty-eight for men, and twenty-five or twenty-six for women. The only dip occurred during the Industrial Revolution. Even in 1930, the mean age for first marriages in this country was still twenty-five for women and twenty-seven for men. Only in the 1970s did it fall to twenty-three and twenty-four. Many people did not marry at all (there was a high spinster rate) and although the majority of the population during the three centuries preceding ours lived in households containing six or more people, only two per cent of households contained twelve or more people (including lodgers and servants) and only one third contained six or more.[2]

The nuclear family has been with us for longer than we think, and so has the spacing of children. What has changed in the West since the turn of the century is the pattern of spacing. Whereas the pre-1900 mother had five or six living children spaced evenly across her fertile phase, the tendency since 1900 has been for her to compress her childbearing into the early years of marriage. During the seventeenth, eighteenth and nineteenth centuries, the span from first marriage to last child was 14.4 years. In the 1950s it was less than 8.5. Before 1800 the mean age for a mother bearing her last child was forty. In the 1880s it was thirty-three, and in the 1920s it was thirty. Add to this the rise in life expectancy, and you find another important difference. Before 1900, mothers could expect to live twenty years after the birth of their last child. After 1900, she could expect to live fifty years. In other words, she would now look foward to thirty or more years without dependent children.[3]

Just as the family has changed in shape, it has changed in meaning. Family historians belonging to the 'sentiments' school describe the family *circa* 1600 as patriarchal and authoritarian. Marriage served an economic function. The duty was to respect and obey rather than to love. The boundaries between the household and the community in which it was situated were permeable, with the result that community ties were often stronger than family ties, and community interference commonplace and accepted. It was only gradually that the home became a haven from the outside world, and privacy, domesticity, romantic love, and ideas about good mothering made the family the child-centred unit we like to think it is today.[4]

As for the actual shape of families, the 'household economics' school of family historians has presented convincing evidence for the theory that it has always been dictated by inheritance and employment opportunities. We in the twentieth century are not the first people ever to plan our families in accordance with our material aspirations. Throughout the ages, families may have adopted 'often unconscious strategies' to maintain a certain standard of living. The problem all families have always faced is the same problem over which we are fretting, i.e. 'the need to ensure enough labour is available to meet current and future needs, while making sure there are not too many mouths to feed.'[5]

The ideal number of children depends on the nature of the work that is open to them. If the parents live on a farm, they'll want plenty of helping hands. If they find themselves involved in an early industry that employs children, they might want even more than before. If child mortality is high, they'll have more children than they expect to survive. If their parents control the property, they'll marry according to their parents' wishes. If they live in a town where it is possible to set up house without dowries or inheritance, and where it makes sense to have children while their earning power is

Fertility is Political

still high, they will follow that strategy. In other words, that imaginary monolith, the head of household with the nine-to-five job and a wife and two children at home, is a configuration that has only ever existed in the tiny pockets of history and suburbia where it was economically feasible.

What *has* changed recently and relatively suddenly is the way in which a family regulates fertility. Or, to put it more bluntly, what the man's domain is, and the means by which he controls the woman who provides the means of reproduction. Forget pregnancy and babies for a minute, and take the long view. Remember: we're talking about the next generation, about the transmission of wealth, genes, and cultural values. In the past, a traditional head of household could not decide exactly who had how many children when, but if he held the purse strings, and if the society he lived in was reasonably patriarchal in its social organisation, he could decide, as head of family, which children to support and which to disinherit, which to call legitimate and which illegitimate. With these sanctions at his disposal, he could feel in control, if not of his fertility, then of the women who implemented it, and the families that resulted.

No longer can he enjoy such peace of mind. According to the French family historian, Donzelot, the erosion of his powers began centuries ago. In *The Policing of Families* (and by policing he means improving, modernising, and streamlining), he describes with admirable Gallic sarcasm the way in which the social anarchy following the French Revolution provided doctors with the opportunity to reform the already tottering patriarchal family by forming an alliance with mothers in the interests of 'hygiene'. By educating the mothers about superior child and health care, doctors gave mothers the ideas and the confidence they needed to strengthen their power base. As their domestic role grew more important, so the role of the patriarchs became less important. But at the same time, the mothers remained beholden to doctors. They were pawns in some very grand plans to improve the quality of the human race. Donzelot quotes one eighteenth-century idealist who recommended founding an institution that would regulate fertility and control vice by combining the functions of a convent, a foundling hospital, and a brothel.[6] Another visionary doctor of the same era, the author of *Le Cité Futur*, recommended a medical tribunal which would examine all citizens between the ages of fifteen and seventeen, and pass them as suitable candidates for procreation, or else defer them for a year, or sterilise them.[7]

It is not recorded what the citizens thought of such measures. That these plans did not come to fruition would seem to indicate that the dreaming doctors met with some resistance. But it is important to remember that eugenics was a discipline with many respectable adherents until Hitler took its premise to the logical extreme.

One very important believer in the 'great white race' was Marie Stopes, who opened the first family planning clinic in this country in 1921 and is sometimes called the mother of the family planning movement. She dedicated her 1918 book, *Wise Parenthood*, 'to all those who wish to see our face grow in strength and beauty.'[8] 'Whatever theory of the transmission of characteristics scientists may ultimately adopt,' she says in her opening chapter, 'there can be little doubt in the minds of rational people that heredity *does* tell, and that children who descend from a double line of healthy and intelligent parents are better equipped to face whatever difficulties in their environment may later arise than are children from unsound stock. . . . We must breed from the physically, morally, and intellectually fit.' Men and women who are 'truly in love' naturally desire children, she says, 'unless they are aware that either is stricken by some inherent weakness or disease which might reappear in the child. Then they must refrain from parenthood out of a sense of duty and pity towards the unborn.'[9] She recommends 'a wise, reasoned and controlled use of the most intimate and sacred functions of the body'[10] and wants each pair of healthy lovers to 'bring forth children for the race, who have the best chance which that pair can give them of health and beauty and happiness. . . . Our race is weakened by an appallingly high percentage of unfit weaklings and diseased individuals. Vicious and feebleminded people reproduce . . . more recklessly and bring forth children who are weakened and handicapped by physical as well as mental warping and weakness.' These monsters overtax the resources of 'the sound and thrifty.... Only children with the chance of attaining strong, beautiful, and intelligent children should be conceived.'[11] She has two sets of standards, always clearly stated. Healthy, intelligent, beautiful people should practise contraception in early marriage, during the first year of each child's life, and after the family has six children. People who are insane, epileptic, alcoholic, who do not have enough food, or whose existing children are 'puny and utterly unsatisfactory' should use contraception all the time.[12] She warns against 'the racial dangers which are so often coincident with illicit love'.[13] 'It seems easy enough,' she concludes, 'to supply the intelligent and careful woman with physiological help; and for the careless, stupid, or feebleminded who persist in producing infants of no value to the state and often only a charge upon it, the right course seems to be sterilisation.'[14]

We can giggle nervously about her glaring prejudices today, but the fact we fail to look in the face is that the family planning movement was founded to produce two results – first, the bettering of conditions for the middle-class woman, and second, to stop social undesirables from reproducing themselves. Today's family planning movement does not adhere to these ideas, but the skeleton of eugenics is there in the cupboard, and, as we shall see in the next chapter, the Marie Stopes approach to fertility control continues to make subtle, disguised appearances in most of our general debates about overpopulation and teenage pregnancy. There may not be programmes specifically set up to keep people of low morals from procreating outside wedlock, or to bar degenerates and misfits from parenthood, but the wish is still there, the aim still expressed, albeit in muted terms. It would be so much better, polite people still murmur in the safety of their own homes, if the races, groups, and types of people who are having too many children 'for their own good' could only be persuaded to make better use of contraception. Professionals working in the family planning field are able to promote that very aim without challenging the sanctity of choice by defining the problem as unwanted pregnancy.

As we pointed out earlier, the term itself is never clearly defined.

It is usually deemed sufficient to state the numbers. It seems to be a given, for example, that there are a million unwanted teenage pregnancies a year in the US, but it is never said how many of these occur within marriages or 'stable relationships' or what criteria the information gatherers have used in order to establish what makes a pregnancy unwanted. It is thought self-evident that an unwanted teenage pregnancy leads directly to dire social problems. The term one concerned psychologist uses is 'Malthusian disaster'.[15] Malthus, you may recall, was the eighteenth-century writer who believed that the poor, if left to their own devices, would reproduce to their natural limits, outstripping the food supply, and were only to be checked by war, disease, and natural disasters. He was the target of Swift's *A Modest Proposal*, which, as you may also remember, suggested that the powers that be could solve the Irish population problem by eating their babies.

So what does all this tell us about the changes in the way families control fertility? The story we usually tell ourselves is that it used to be the woman who made the decisions within the very strict limits set by her patriarchal husband, and that now, thanks to improved birth control, better educational and economic opportunities, and relaxed social sanctions, she is free to make her fertility decisions without getting permission from anyone. But if you consider the model proposed by Donzelot – the idea that women were first able to improve their lot by forming a pact with doctors – you can begin to see that the sequence of events leading to our current liberated state might be a good deal more complicated. We can trace many of our gains in this country back to an old and always uneasy feminist–medical alliance. From the very beginning of the women's movement, there has existed the conviction that women need to be freed from the yoke of perpetual motherhood if they are to advance themselves. Doctors have provided the wherewithal to make this possible, and in so doing they have turned fertility from women's business into medical business. This is not the same as saying that doctors control fertility: their role is persuasive. They are teachers and counsellors, not judges. In this country at least, they are meant not just to leave the final decisions to women, but also to respect these opinions. Of course there are, in practice, consistent abuses of this principle. But it is important to remember that the result of the alliance between the woman and the doctor remains more or less the same, regardless. It continues to have the same effect which Donzelot detected in post-revolutionary France: it undermines the power of the patriarch, now better known as the husband, the partner, the 'child's father' and sometimes even 'the sperm donor'.

So there we have it. That's what has changed. After millennia of procreating under the ever watchful, punitive eyes of the patriarch–inseminator, now finally, thanks to the intervention of doctors, the woman is behind the steering wheel, the deposed patriarch in a sulk in the passenger seat next to her. Nobody seems too interested in him for the time being. The eyes of society are on the woman. The question on all our lips is: does she know how to drive? Remember – if she doesn't, she can endanger the safety as well as the quality of the next generation. Never mind that she, too, is a creature of tradition, and will, no matter how radical her plans or irresponsible her appearance, probably share our sentimental view of the family-as-haven. Tolerance is hard to maintain when it comes to other people's fertility. Today's liberated woman must not be left to her own devices – we cannot afford to live the mistakes she'll create if she is permitted to grow into her new powers naturally. She must be made aware that she is now in control of a very dangerous machine. Before we can allow her to travel about unsupervised, she must receive proper instruction.

We like to think of sex education as a new phenomenon. Certainly we have moved way beyond the mysterious wilderness of birds, bees, rabbits and lampposts. Most people working in the field today know that euphemisms confuse rather than instruct, and that the didactic, authoritarian approach can be counterproductive. There is a growing emphasis on communication, affective education, and follow-up. In other words, the student is not to be addressed as a foot soldier, there to receive and carry out specific marching orders, but as a future decision-maker, there to be shown how to develop judgement, take the long view, form strategies, carry out negotiations, and make adjustments and compromises, so as to better achieve that most exalted of negative goals, the avoidance of pregnancy.

In other words, it's a different set of means designed to achieve the same end. Take off the protective packaging and what sex educators are saying today is the same thing your mother told you after giving you the facts of life while she was ironing: 'Don't do anything stupid.' The name of the game is the suppression of fertility. In the old days, the only way to make sure that young, unattached girls didn't get pregnant at the drop of a hat was to promote and safeguard the virtue of virginity. Now, with the advent of contraception, virginity is no longer the point of no return. Women can have sex without getting pregnant. Public interest has therefore shifted from a woman's 'morals' to her use of birth control. Sex education exists to make sure she knows how to use it properly. In this sense, it is taking up the mantle once worn by parents, religious leaders, and guardians of public morality. The basic message remains the same: early babies, in other words, babies born before you're a fully established adult, can ruin lives. Sex educators are as committed as ever to spreading the contraceptive mentality, with the result that most of us in our fertile phase today – even those of us who had the benefit of enlightened instruction – tend to associate contraception with obedience, and have come to understand fertility as a force to be repressed rather than as a force to be understood and managed in different ways at different times in our lives.

We believe it is this contraceptive mentality that makes us such willing pawns in the game of fertility politics. All the speakers in the fertility debate are concerned with controlling that wild card – the female body. All the speakers express their views by using the female body as a metaphor. For the doctor, it is a beautiful, perfectible machine; for the traditionalist, a vessel; for the feminist, a control centre; for the family planner, a beautiful, perfectible machine that can, with the proper instruction, become a control centre so socially responsible it could pass for a vessel. There is a place for these metaphors, and a place for debates about who controls the next generation. The problem now is that little effort is made to distinguish between the real bodies of real women trying to make real decisions, and the metaphorical bodies of fertility politics. The body imagery of the latter haunts the real woman as she exercises her right to choose. It confuses the issues – and makes clear-headed thinking very difficult.

To illustrate this problem, let us imagine a woman who has received the best, most comprehensive fertility preparation on offer. Let us also assume that her attitude and her intentions are similarly beyond reproach. She is at the beginning of her fertile life, and she is determined to negotiate all its challenges responsibly. How does she feel as she surveys the paths that are open to her?

She feels pulled in opposite directions by competing rights and obligations. On the one hand, she believes that she has earned the right to decide if and when she has children, and also to determine what size family is right for her. On the other hand, she feels a certain responsibility about world population levels. She therefore can't let herself be too greedy. As a woman she treasures her rights too much to let a man set the fertility agenda; by the same token, she would hate to impose *her* fertility agenda on a man. Where is the golden mean? And what type of partnership is she looking for? She isn't sure what she does expect from the father of any child she might have. Would she want him to share the child-care? To provide financial support? Even if she doesn't, would he be justified in vetoing a plan for a child because he didn't want her to give up *her* job? It's her right to have a child alone, of course, if that's what she decides is best for her, but is it best for the child? Why does she want children at all, if motherhood is going to put her at such a big disadvantage in the workplace?

If all she had to do was to grapple with these dilemmas in the privacy of her own home, it would be hard enough. Unhappily, these are questions that have trickled down to her from the desperately unresolved public debates about freedom of the individual versus global obligations, about motherhood as privilege versus motherhood as burden, about maternal rights versus fetal rights. . . . She will find herself fiercely lobbied.

How does this intrusive attention make her feel? If you've never found yourself in this position, imagine that you are the driver of a dodgem car, a dodgem car you must take care not to crash as you struggle to the other side of a rink crowded with countless other confused and meandering dodgem car drivers. It is all you can do to stay out of their way, so what are you to make of the throngs of hecklers on the sidelines? Each one is criticising your driving. Each one has a different idea of what you ought to do next. But how are you supposed to concentrate if you pause to listen to even one of them? At a certain point, you will put your foot on the brake and cry, 'Stop telling me what to do! Let *ME* decide!'

'It's my right to choose!' you insist, but, even as you assert yourself, you will be repeating a line that has been fed to you, a line that is only correct up to a point. The woman's right to choose is the cornerstone of enlightened sex education, family planning, and medical care, but the fact remains that such services exist not to protect individual rights at any cost, but to serve the public good by training individuals to make decisions in a socially responsible way. In other words, even the most personal fertility decision wears a social face and is, in fact, a social decision. And when we make a socially responsible decision, all we're really doing is internalising a social imperative.

It would be hard enough if the social imperatives *vis-à-vis* fertility were clear cut. But fertility being the political hot potato it is, there's no consensus about what is right. There's always some heckler out there to convince you that whatever you did, you were wrong, with the result that almost all of us feel like walking wounded.

Add to that our own assessment of our poor qualifications. Standards for parenthood go way up the moment it ceases to be a condition that either happens or doesn't, that one grows into and accepts, and becomes a matter of conscious choice. Listen to this list of questions from a pamphlet entitled 'Am I Parent Material?' provided by the British Organisation of Non-Parents:

What sort of a parent would I be?

1. Do I like children? Have I had enough contact with babies? toddlers? teenagers?
2. Do I have enough love to give a child? Can I express

affection easily? How much love would I expect my child to give me?

3. Would I have the patience to bring up a child? Can I tolerate noise and confusion? Can I deal with disrupted routines? And not just by babies, but by toddlers, children and moody teenagers?

4. How do I handle anger? Would I batter my baby if I lost my temper?

5. What do I know about discipline and freedom? Would I be too strict? Too lenient? Would I get upset if things weren't perfect?

6. What kind of relationship do I have with my own parents? Would I want to have the same relationship with my children?

7. How much would I worry about my child? Would I be overprotective?

8. What if my decision to have a child turns out to have been wrong for me?

Would a child fit into my way of life?

1. Would a baby interfere with apprenticeship or education plans? . . .

2. Would I have to give up interests and activities I feel are important to me?

3. Could I handle children and work? Do I have plenty of energy at the end of the day or am I tired?

4. Am I able to support a child? . . .

5. Do I live in a neighbourhood where I would like to bring up a child? If not, would I be willing to move?

6. Would I be willing and happy to restrict my social life? Would I miss lost leisure time and privacy?

7. Would I be prepared to be a single parent if my partner left or died?

8. Would I be happy and willing to devote a great part of my life, at least sixteen years, to be responsible for a child? And be concerned about my child's welfare for the rest of my life?

What do I expect to gain from the experience of being a parent?

1. Am I happy playing Monopoly all afternoon – even though I am bored after one game – or leaving the Zoo after ten minutes – even though it cost us £5 to get in?

2. Would I have a baby to prove to others that I am grown up?

3. Would I want my child to be like me? Would I be willing to adopt a child?
4. What would I do if my child had ideas and beliefs different from mine? How different?
5. Would I expect my child to do all the things I wished I had done?
6. Would I expect my child to keep me from being lonely in my old age? How?
7. Would I expect a baby to make my marriage complete?
8. Would I feel strongly about wanting a boy or a girl? What if I didn't get the one I wanted? . . .

Anyone who already has children will read this list of questions and be reminded of problems and surprises they have faced in the past, are grappling with now, or anticipate meeting in the future. But this will almost always be followed by a shrug of the shoulders, and a comment along the lines of 'So what? These things are just part of life.' The authors of the questionnaire are right in trying to get beyond the 'perfect picture' that so many prospective parents have in mind when they make their decisions: all the problems the questions suggest are not just valid, but will affect almost everyone. But to suggest that anyone could ever be ready for the challenge – to suggest that you must become a parenthood spiritually before attempting it physically – is to make any decision about childbearing far heavier, far, far more significant than it needs to be.

When we decide to have, or not to have, a child these days, we are – even when we are sensible enough to try not to – taking an ethical position on the great debates of our day; we are formulating a policy; we are making a statement; we are putting ourselves forward for the exalted state of parenthood. We are confirming our place in the scheme of things, or else challenging it. The actual child who may result from such cerebral manoeuvres hardly even enters into it. If babies could rise fully formed like Aphrodite out of Poseidon's shoulder, then perhaps everything would be all right. Unhappily they cannot get started without the proper management, and the co-operation, of not one, but two bodies. We have already pointed out how ill-equipped we are to manage this dark and mysterious force, and also how very uncooperative our body can be when we issue it orders. The result is that we often find ourselves pregnant without a plan, or else not pregnant in spite of a plan. In the first scenario we will be aghast at our own (overestimated) power. In the second scenario, we will be aghast at our (again, overestimated) impotence. These feelings will have a big effect on the choices we make next. Although the words 'child' and 'baby' will come up frequently in our deliberations, they will be largely symbolic and usually secondary: our first job will be to do whatever needs to be done to get 'the situation back under control'.

What we are looking at, then, is engorged decision-making, in which a postulated child provokes not just practical questions, but an exhaustive soul-search about love, money, sex, ambition, politics, truth, and even beauty. It is something almost all of us are engaged in. It doesn't matter if we are making blinkered plans way in advance, or if we are continually making the decision to defer the big decision, or if we just 'let things happen' and face the very loud and accusing music in the event of an accident. These are just different responses to the same sphinx – to the insoluble, unbudgeable dilemma that the decision to have, or not to have a child has become today.

CHAPTER FOURTEEN

THE DOWNGRADED PARENT, THE PERFECTIBLE CHILD AND THE SPECTRE OF EUGENICS

'There are times when I would look across the room and think, "Why is this woman sitting in my house asking me how much I drink, and how many books I read a month?" ' The speaker is Maggie, now the mother of two young adopted children. Their first adoption was, they thought at the time, gruelling – there were constant visits from social workers, and because they were working with a Catholic charity, her husband, a lapsed Catholic, had to go back into the Church. 'He had to start going to confession. We even had to get married again. The second time was easier for us because the first time we always felt like they were trying to catch us out. We had a much better social worker the second time round. She was very supportive, the mother of eight. But I don't know if we would have made it through that one if we didn't have the confidence we got from already having a child at home.

'The first surprise was that we had to apply all over again – fill out all the same forms about how many primary schools we had been to and so on, and then they worked out that somehow we had slipped through the net the first time round and missed the six seminars for adoptive parents. The bias of these seminars was that the child was most important, the biological parent was next most important, and you, the adoptive parents, were least important. We were very upset about this. They practically told us we counted for little more than baby-sitters. When we complained to the social worker, she explained that the bias was because social workers spent so much time picking up the pieces for people who hadn't been told they were adopted until they were adults. She kept saying we were better able to cope because we'd been through it, but there was a social worker for the baby, too, and she put us through the mill, too, by exposing us to the pain of the biological mother, a very brave and mature seventeen-year-old. I admire this woman, the biological mother, for wanting to face up to things and meet us and make sure she was putting the baby into good hands, but the social worker got too involved. And then there were appalling foster parents who had never fostered before . . . still, we were very lucky. It's so unusual to get nice, healthy babies, and now we have two . . . considering we're fako Catholics, we got a very good deal.'

You listen to this woman and you think, 'How unfair'. It's clear at a moment's glance that she is an able and dedicated mother. Not that we would want adoption officers making snap decisions based on instincts. But does the vetting have to be that humiliating, that thorough? Do the standards have to be that inflexible and narrow? Why, if a couple has adopted one child successfully, do they have to start from scratch again when they apply for a second?

Those are the questions that occur to the outsider. But even adoptive parents are usually keen to make clear that they see the point of regulations. Maggie herself contrasted the ordeal she and her husband went through with the experience of an American couple who attempted a private adoption with no intermediaries by putting an advertisement in a newspaper. They liked the sound of one woman who got in touch with them and went so far as to pay all her expenses, including her phone bill. It turned out to be a con. But they didn't give up. 'The woman told me that the con had felt like having a miscarriage and being raped at the same time. She says she's given up work and spends all her time sitting by the phone waiting for the right person to get in touch. When I heard that story, I said to myself, "Bring back the social workers!" '

Another woman we spoke to, who was able to adopt a newborn baby in South America with very few formalities, said that the lack of intermediaries worked to her advantage because they got the baby soon after birth and were able to make a quick and graceful adjustment to parenthood. But she doesn't recommend this as a

The Downgraded Parent

system, because it would mean that a baby could end up with anybody, leading to terrible abuses. Social workers in this country make a similar argument against foreign adaptation. As one said to us: 'Inappropriate couples find themselves with irreparably damaged children. Devastation can follow.'

And with it, intervention. As Toinette, another adoptive mother told us: 'When I made the obvious objection about our being so very carefully vetted, while there were plenty of women living on the same street who could have children whenever they wanted without any vetting whatsoever, the social worker said, "Oh, don't you worry. We'll be catching up with them later." '

That is precisely what most of us forget when we talk about fertility as body politics, and consequently, as something we can both own and control. We might be able to decide when and if to exercise our fertility rights, but we do not own and so cannot have unchallenged control over the children that might result. As much as we might complain about insensitive health visitors, intrusive teachers and malevolent social workers, few of us today would wish on ourselves a society where parents were free to be unexamined tyrants.

So, yes, we want children to be guaranteed certain protections. We want standards to be set for parents, and we want children who are abused and neglected to be removed from parental custody. We want to make sure children who are wards of the state are placed in 'good homes'. But the question is – who is setting the standards? What do officials mean when they say someone is suitable for parenthood?

It emerged recently that there is a trend to turn down smokers who apply to adopt foster children. The reason for this is that children must be protected from the dangers of passive smoking. The media response to this new item was: But how ludicrous! Think of all the "natural" children who are exposed to the still not fully substantiated dangers of passive smoking. It's not fair to apply such impossibly high standards to prospective adopters when "natural" parents can do as they please.

Yes, we say, but it's not true that natural parents are judged by a different set of standards. 'Natural' parents might be more difficult to control, but we are all measured up to the same ideal model. And we find the purest expression of this ideal coming from the mouths of adoption officers.

'A really, really good parent does not blow smoke in her child's face.' So speaks a health official, adding afterwards, 'Although of course that is not the be all and end all.' The problem, in our view, is that public agencies refer back too often to principles of hygiene, both physical and moral, that echo the mottoes of eugenics.

Look, for example, at the vetting that patients seeking fertility treatment must undergo. Few of us would want such services to be provided to 'just anyone'. The new gender selection clinics are a case in point – it doesn't take long to imagine how such a service could be (and is already being) abused, especially in cultures where sons are preferred to daughters. But why does a woman seeking IVF at a superior, non-profit clinic, have to be in a stable relationship, and what counts for stable? Why must she have no history of mental illness? Does a depression or a one-time visit to a psychiatrist count as mental illness? Why must the applicant prove her eagerness to have a child?

But most of all – why are we leaving the decision to the doctor? Why aren't we all contributing to the debate on what our current standard of parenthood ought to be – instead of leaving it to public officials and then grumbling about their insensitivity and lack of understanding?

Why, instead of trying to figure out what side we are on, don't we examine the terms of the debate? We cite as an example the recent US controversy about Norplant. Norplant is a device that consists of small capsules the size of match sticks that can be inserted under the skin of a woman's arm, where they release a hormone called progestin for about five years and thus inhibit ovulation. A number of states are considering giving cash incentives to welfare mothers who have the device inserted. Others are considering punitive measures for welfare mothers who refuse it, and there have been some proposals that Norplant implantations be forced on people in extreme cases. Isobel Sawhill, a senior fellow at the left-leaning

The Downgraded Parent

Washington think-tank, the Urban Institute, has gone so far as to propose that all girls in the US be provided with the implant at puberty. 'It could protect nearly a million teenagers from unwelcome pregnancies each year,' she has said.[1]

Look at the way she defines the problem. Unwelcome pregnancy, as far as she is concerned, is a disease, and so best managed in the same way as a flu epidemic. You would think that the opposition would question this assumption, and ask, too, for more details about the million tragic pregnancies. What ages are the mothers? To what socio-economic groups do they belong? How many are thirteen, and how many nineteen? Clearly, all the pregnancies are unwelcome to the public, but how many were unwelcome to the mothers themselves? And how unwelcome?

But no. The right-leaning think-tank, the Family Research Council, was only concerned that such a measure might lead to greater promiscuity, and therefore moral and social decay. 'You need to make people change their conduct, not just accept that sex on demand is given.'[2]

Maybe so, but by failing to question this apparently universal principle – that all teenage pregnancies are tragic and that all teenage parents are unsuitable – we drift closer and closer to the idea that people need to meet certain age and hygiene requirements before gaining the right to parenthood.

It may sound preposterous, but, as we have already mentioned, there is, even today, a serious public discussion going on about the physical prerequisites for parenthood as screening methods for undesirable traits become cheaper and more effective. At the very least, insurance companies might deny coverage for the undesirable gene-carrying adult or the correctly screened but unaborted imperfect child, and the health service could deny care.

At present, we have amniocentesis, Chorionic Villus Sample (CVS) and sophisticated blood tests to detect or determine the likelihood of Down's syndrome, cystic fibrosis, and neural tube defects. Soon we will be able to screen fetuses for cancer, hypercholesterolaemia and Alzheimer's disease. While there has been a fair amount of responsible debate about the ethics of all this, it has not been so loud as to prevent some experts in the field from crowing about exciting new trends in research, using terminology that ought to have gone out of style with Hitler.

Here is what Timothy Chard, Clinical Director of Obstetrics and Gynaecology at St Bartholomew's Hospital Medical College is reported to have said recently to a postgraduate meeting of the Royal College of Obstetricians and Gynaecologists: 'We are in the middle of a revolution in terms of the elimination of imperfections. This has been brought about by advances in embryo biopsy, the measurement of chemicals in maternal blood, and ultrasound imaging. We are already most of the way there in eliminating the three major causes of abnormality. . . . Tests for the more minor conditions will follow in the next ten years. A near perfect child will be available to every parent who has access to the technology – about twenty per cent of the world population – by early next century.'

He went on to distinguish between the 'perfect' child and the 'superior' child. 'The former is one that is healthy and normal and the latter is one with health, beauty, and brains.' The superior child, he assured his audience, was not going to be possible for the 'foreseeable, long-term future'.[3]

The main concern of the audience seems to have been the 'slash and burn' mentality which relies on terminations upon discovery of a problem. The professor's response was that it was important to do more work to prevent these conditions from developing at all. What no one seems to have questioned was the pursuit of the perfect, defect-free child, the ideal of quantifiable brains, beauty, and health. Why do we suddenly have no room for imperfection? Why have we forgotten that one person's imperfection is another person's grain in the oyster? What about traits that are both strengths and weakness? And, most important, who is writing the definitions?

The problem, as we see it, is that we are all – not just Professor Chard – talking about the imaginary child. Which, by definition, is perfect. Dreams don't have flaws, at least not to their owners. There is nothing wrong with imaginary children – except when you forget that they are not real.

And yet we have forgotten – or at least we don't remind ourselves often enough – that just as fertility is the *potential* to have children, so we make our fertility *choices* in the abstract. Even the unfortunate woman who is deterred from entering an abortion clinic by Rescue America's reprehensible billboards featuring photographs of mangled fetuses is responding to a symbol, not a real baby.

And because fertility is a power that lives primarily in the land of the hypothetical, we fail to see the terms 'perfect', 'suitable' and 'wanted' as the dangerous road signs they are. If we continue not to do so, the age of personal fertility choice could lead to the age of regulated procreation. If we allow eugenics into polite discourse through the back door, we will be giving up our natural right to parenthood. And if we do, it won't just be the fault of the doctors and researchers and legislators. It will also be because we have become too guilty, or too preoccupied with the minutiae of fertility consumerism to defend our own turf.

Our counterproposal? To reframe the debate so that we can all participate in it. To move away from pro-life, pro-choice polar oppositions and either/or questions into more practical discussions about limits. How much freedom, how much supervision is right for a particular society at a particular time? What has to happen before those lines are re-drawn? How much should we be examining, and questioning, the words we use to describe parents, babies, and families? How much are our social prejudices clouding our judgement?

We would like to propose a broader understanding of fertility as something that begins in the body but does not end there. Because fertility concerns the creation and formation of the next generation, it concerns us all. There is a place for fertility politics, and a place for medical fertility, but we as individuals must reserve our basic rights and privileges.

How? By ceasing to judge ourselves so harshly for our failure to be effective corporate decision-makers, and interpreting our behaviour instead by the kinder, more flexible, and less value-laden model of the calculated risk-taker. By participating in the political debate about fertility without letting these large, as yet unresolved questions confuse the fertility dilemmas we face in our personal lives. And last but not least, by standing back and looking at the term 'fertility control' and figuring out exactly what this means in our brave new world of reproductive technology and personal choice.

Ask the woman on the street what it means and she'll probably say it means contraception and abortion. Query her on abortion, and if this doesn't prompt her to speak on the subject of the sanctity of life, she will probably say something along the lines of abortion being a necessary evil, a fall-back method without which no woman could be guaranteed self-determination. Pressed to speak about the anti-abortion movement, this woman would probably say that in her view, all the anti-abortion people want is to push woman back into the traditional family and rob her of her new-found autonomy. What she is unlikely to add is that if you take the broader definition of fertility, as something that begins in the body but also concerns the formation of the next generation, the state that legalises abortion is also in the position to rob women of their new-found autonomy – by encouraging those people deemed unsuitable as parents to have abortions, while putting the opposite kind of pressure on people who appear suitable. This certainly doesn't happen in this country in any kind of systematic way, but where doctors, counsellors, teachers, parents and so on allow their social prejudices about suitability and unsuitability for parenthood to intervene, the result is all too often an abortion which is not an act of free choice but an act of obedience.

Fertility control, in other words, does not necessarily mean that the woman is in control. If we want to retain any degree of autonomy, it is important to know when and where other, larger social forces have vested interests in the types of choices we are making. We need to know what kinds of fertility control we want to have for ourselves, what we don't mind sharing, and what we want to have no part in.

Our definition of fertility control is 'anything that we do to prevent birth, to regulate conception, or to optimise the chances of a "normal" child.' This is an umbrella that covers everything from pre-conceptual care through family planning and abortion to fertility treatment and genetic screening. When you look at all the choices together, they beg the questions – how much control *do* I want to have over my unborn offspring? How much quality control is too much quality control? How will I feel when the day comes that no woman can see her pregnancy as confirmed until she has passed twenty or more weeks' worth of genetic screening hurdles? How much control over such matters am I willing to cede to others, and how much would I prefer to leave to fate?

The answers will be different for each person – and change for each person often over the course of a lifetime. But just as informed choices are choices you make without blinkers, and in full awareness of what fertility control implies, so are informed choices based on a detailed understanding of the medical fertility controls on offer – how they work on your body, and what their advantages and disadvantages are. In the next three chapters, we hope to provide the calculated risk-taker with this information. But first, let's look at how the body works without them.

CHAPTER FIFTEEN

HOW FERTILE ARE WE?

'It's ticking away.' When a woman says this about her 'biological clock', what she usually means is that she's afraid she might be running out of time. She's thirty-four or thirty-five and still she's not comfortably off, still she hasn't found a man she would want to be the father of her children. Her worries are practical and worldly. She still assumes that all she has to do to conceive is to stop taking contraception. Her ability to reproduce is not an issue worthy of discussion – largely thanks to the mechanical image that dominates her understanding of her fertility.

The biological clock, as most people understand it, is something that winds up fast, stays ticking absolutely accurately for thirty years, and stops abruptly. This is not to say there aren't rumours abounding about misleading warranties and defective parts. There is always some expert somewhere who is trying to prove that the fertility rate amongst women over thirty – particularly women over thirty with career ambitions – is on the decline. Even where the evidence is clearly flimsy, the very suggestion of an 'infertility epidemic' instils fear in the hearts of women who have deferred their plans for a family. Perhaps this is why media scares about fertility prompt them to talk about their biological clocks ticking louder, instead of begging some questions about terminology that ought to have been obvious.

What, after all, is a fertility rate? Fertility is a potential, not an event. It doesn't depend on the health and age of one person, but of two. How can it be quantified? Are we counting conceptions, pregnancies, births? Sperm, couples or individuals? What's the difference between a birth rate and a fertility rate? Why is it always women who matter in fertility statistics? What about men? And how about the term 'infertility rate'? In *Backlash*, Susan Faludi did a heroic job of demolishing the so-called scientific studies that scaremongers had used to convince American women over thirty that they might never be able to conceive – and yet she herself uses this mysterious term 'infertility rate'.[1] Which is? The rate at which women fail to conceive? At what ages? After how many months? Under what clinical conditions? At which times of the month, how frequently, and (bearing in mind that thirty per cent of all infertility problems in couples are traced solely to the male) with the help of donors with what baseline sperm count?

When people – and particularly journalists – discuss fertility rates, they rarely say what they mean by the term. This is a shame, because it means something different to every researcher. The most responsible definition – and the one that turns up most frequently in family planning literature – is 'the number of children a woman bears in the course of her lifetime'. If this is the yardstick, then a fertility rate will tell you quite a bit about demographic patterns – i.e. how families choose to space their children – and next to nothing about the ability of women in specific age brackets to bear children. And *less* than zero about men.

We would like to urge you away from the never-never land of lies, statistics and biological clocks, and propose a more complex understanding of the specific processes which make it possible for us to reproduce. To give a rough overview before we start: in a man we are talking about the production – and delivery – of the right quality and number of sperm. In a woman we are talking about the production and proper release of eggs, the ability to receive, protect and channel sperm, the successful implantation of any fertilised eggs in the lining of the uterus, and the ability to sustain a pregnancy. All of these processes are fragile. As well as being influenced by age and state of health, they are quick to register changes in mood, diet, sleep patterns, temperature, environment, weight, medication and stress level. If you had a clock that acted like that, would you ever believe anything you saw on its face? If you insist on a mechanical metaphor for measuring fertility, a far better one would be a seismograph. But better still would be to throw out these 'image crutches' and try to understand what's really going on in our bodies.

Let's start by defining the boundaries. When does a person become fertile? The answer for boys is usually vague and involves a description of the various physical changes that occur at puberty. The answer for girls is usually 'the first menstruation' – although this is, technically speaking, the culmination of a long series of events including a growth spurt. It is generally assumed that any girl who has menstruated is able to conceive, but a girl's early cycles are often anovulatory, i.e. without ovulation, irregular, and more easily affected by stress and travelling than they will be later on. Many girls are not told about their cervical secretions and so see them as an abnormal discharge. They also tend to assume that anything other than a twenty-eight-day cycle makes them abnormal. This fear is often inadvertently reinforced by sex educators and doctors, who cling to this magic number with surprising tenacity. In fact, even those who achieve the Golden Mean will rarely do so right away.

Regular menstruation does not automatically mean regular ovulation, and regular ovulation does not automatically imply fertility. A woman's reproductive processes build up slowly, take time to work together efficiently. They remain relatively stable up until the age of thirty-five or thereabouts, and then go into a gradual decline until the age of forty, after which fertility in most women falls off more rapidly. Again, this does not mean that a woman setting out to have children after forty will run into trouble. It simply means that she may be ovulating less regularly – first once in every two cycles, then once in every three, four or five – and that even if she does ovulate, there is greater likelihood that the other processes leading up to and following conception might be faulty or out of sync. Or, to put it another way, if all the women in the world were to decide to begin their families after the age of forty, the birth rate would plummet – just as it would soar if all women were to start their families while they were in their early twenties.

A woman may be less likely to become pregnant after forty than she would have been under similar circumstances ten or twenty years earlier – but she cannot be sure she will not conceive until after the menopause. The menopause means the cessation of menstruation. This can only be said to have happened for certain if a woman under the age of fifty has had no periods for two years and a woman over fifty has had no periods for one year. For some women, the menopause can happen as early as age thirty-nine or forty, especially in women who smoke, while for others it will be the mid-fifties. It is not known if the late onset of menstruation implies a late menopause, although family patterns may be indicative. What happened to your mother and your aunts and your grandmother is what's likely to happen to you. The challenge of the century, therefore, is to get them to talk to you about it.

When do men stop being fertile? Again, the answers are vague and quickly move beyond physiological matters like erections and sperm counts to the *Guinness Book of Records*. Suffice it to say that while most men run into technical difficulties such as impotence much earlier, it is not unknown for some men in their eighties and nineties to father children.

Females are born with their full complement of eggs, most of which they go on to lose gradually through a process called atresia. A female fetus has about seven million eggs at five months gestation. By birth this will have been reduced to two million, and by puberty 400,000.[2] Men, on the other hand, produce sperm continuously from puberty until the end of their fertile years.

Compared to the female reproductive system, the male reproductive system works in a fairly straightforward way. It is directed by two 'messenger' hormones from the pituitary gland – the same two hormones, incidentally, that direct women's reproductive systems. Follicle-stimulating hormone stimulates the seminiferous tubules inside the testicles to produce sperm, while luteinising hormone stimulates other specialised cells in the testes, called Leydig cells, to produce the hormone, testosterone. Testosterone not only determines male sexual characteristics, but also helps in the production of sperms. It takes sixty days for germ cells (immature sperm) to become spermatozoa (mature sperm), and then another ten to fourteen days for them to travel from the tightly coiled and packed seminiferous tubules into larger ducts which lead to a larger tube called the epidymis and then to the vas deferens. As they pass through the epidymis (which would be six feet long if uncoiled), they slowly acquire motility, or the ability to move forward by themselves. By the time they reach the vas deferens (the even thicker tube that most men can feel in their scrotum) they are fully formed and ready to fertilise an egg.

Continuing along the same channel into the penis, we have the ejaculatory duct, which will also be supplied by the seminal vesicle, the producer of some of the seminal fluid which will carry and nourish the sperm. The ejaculatory duct leads through the prostate into the urethra. When a man ejaculates, the muscles at the base of his penis pump out between one and six millilitres of seminal fluid. This fluid will contain between one hundred and three hundred million sperm, only a tiny fraction of which will survive the journey through the vagina, the cervix and the uterus into the fallopian tubes, where they may or may not find an egg waiting to be fertilised.[3]

With that awesome thought, we'll return to the finite world of female cycles. So far we've established that these cycles go on for about thirty years, with the very first cycles sometimes being anovulatory; that they tend to last twenty-eight days each (with cycles as short as twenty days and cycles as long as forty-two days not entirely uncommon), and that the various processes occurring during the cycle which permit conception and pregnancy work together most efficiently during the early to middle years of the fertile phase, and somewhat less so during the later years. What we'd like to do now is look at these processes in the order that they occur in a 'normal' cycle, and while we do so, we'd like you to remember that the reproductive system does not operate in isolation. It is regulated and controlled by stimulating messenger hormones from the brain.

The traditional way of measuring a cycle is by counting from the first day of the your last period. If you tell a doctor you are pregnant, that is the first piece of information you'll be asked to give. Although it is not always possible to extrapolate from that the exact date of ovulation and/or conception, it is a useful indicator. But it's not really right. The actual cycle begins on the day *after* your last period. The real reason we keep our records differently is because the beginning of a period is an obvious, clear event, whereas the end is both hard to define and harder to remember.

For clarity's sake, we'll abide with the traditionalists. The average period goes on for five or six days, although longer periods are common in some women. During the latter part of the period, hormones start being released under the influence of the pituitary gland. The first hormone is oestrogen, which stimulates the growth of follicles on the ovary. As each follicle grows, the egg or the ovum inside the follicle matures, with one follicle maturing faster than the others. Now the brain produces a surge of luteinising hormone, which causes the most mature follicle to rupture, releasing the egg. This event is called ovulation.

We tend to think of the uterus as a stagnant organ sitting in the lower pelvis. In fact, the fallopian tubes are mobile. They have feathery endings that waft back and forth waiting to catch a released ovum and gather it into the tubes. There have been scans done of women who have had one fallopian tube removed to show the remaining tube sweeping right across the pelvis to pick up an ovum from the other ovary. This happens because they're highly sensitive to the chemicals being released. The lining of the inner surface of the tubes is also very sensitive. The cells contain very fine little hair-like structures called cilia that move together in one direction to waft the egg along the fallopian tube. These cilia can be easily damaged by infection. If damage occurs to the tubes, the egg will not waft through them fast enough. That is why women with damaged (but still patent, or hollow) fallopian tubes are more likely to have ectopic pregnancies. An ectopic pregnancy occurs when a fertilised egg does not reach the uterus and implants into the lining of the fallopian tube and starts to grow. This is a serious situation and requires surgery urgently because the fallopian tube is likely to rupture, resulting in severe bleeding.

Fertilisation, if it occurs, will take place in the outer third of the fallopian tube – *not* in the uterus. And when is the window of opportunity?

Most of us have been taught that it happens 'in the middle of the month'. For some people, this means a fortnight into the cycle. For others – the ones who were listening in biology class – it means between days twelve and sixteen of a twenty-eight-day cycle (but what about a twenty-six- or a thirty-day cycle?). Some romantics persist in believing, incorrectly, that it is a very pleasurable act of intercourse which releases the egg from the ovary, while for one happy optimist we spoke to, fertilisation occurs if and only if the egg bursts out of the ovary and the sperm shoots into the uterus at precisely the same moment.

In fact, the egg is available for fertilisation for about twelve hours, while the sperm involved can normally be capable of fertilising an ovum for about three days following intercourse. (And it will be only one of those original hundreds of millions of sperms – at the moment an egg has become fertilised by one sperm, it changes chemically to prevent other sperm from penetrating it. If more than one sperm penetrates the ovum simultaneously, the resulting fertilised egg will have too many chromosomes, and if it implants it will almost certainly result in an early miscarriage.)

Ovulation will not necessarily occur on the same day in every cycle. If fraternal twins are in the offing, ovulation will occur more than once during a single cycle, the second ovulation occurring within twenty-four hours of the first. One important thing to bear in mind is that if a cycle is irregular, it is usually because the length of the first half of the cycle – the part of the cycle preceding ovulation – is varying in length – often in response to external factors such as stress and diet. Some women feel a pain – Mittelschmerz – when they ovulate, while others recognise the change in cervical secretions, but for most of us ovulation is an event that is hard to predict.

The ovum will take between sixty and seventy hours to waft down the fallopian tube. The fertilised egg will then try to implant itself into the uterine wall if the environment is conducive. It takes about nine days from the release of the egg until full implantation. (Some recent studies indicate that forty per cent, and perhaps even as many as sixty per cent of all fertilised eggs fail to make this transition and so do not result in pregnancy.) Meanwhile, the empty follicle on the ovary under the influence of luteinising hormone, produces progesterone, the hormone that will sustain the pregnancy in its early stages. If this mechanism is faulty for some reason, then there will not be enough progesterone to sustain full implantation. This is why some women with short luteal phases have problems in conceiving.

If pregnancy does not occur, then the empty follicle shrivels up and stops producing progesterone. The lining of the womb, which had already started building itself up for a possible fertilised egg under the influence of oestrogen, now can no longer sustain itself and so is shed, resulting in the bleeding we call the period.

And how do sperm make their journey from the vagina? A lot depends on the secretion from the cervix (the neck of the uterus). By secretion, we mean liquid secreted by glands in the cervix. This varies in appearance and elasticity according to the phase in the cycle. In the first half of the cycle, under the influence of oestrogen, the secretion changes from being thick and sticky to being crystal clear and stretchy like the white of an uncooked egg. Under a microscope it dries to produce beautiful ferning patterns. This clear secretion has channels in it like swimming lanes in a pool. Healthy sperm that can swim straight continue forward through the secretion, while unhealthy sperm with malformed tails or broken necks get caught in the sides of the channels. The alkaline cervical secretion protects the sperm from the hostile, acidic environment of the vagina. Those that swim through to the cervix often rest in small pockets in the wall of the cervix called crypts for a couple of days before swimming into the friendlier environment of the uterus and beyond. Another term for the oestrogen-derived secretion is 'fertile mucus' – a term we have noticed puts people off and makes them less inclined to find out more about it.

Under the influence of progesterone, which is the hormone that replaces oestrogen for the second half of a normal cycle, cervical secretions become thick and sticky. They form a plug in the cervix that is impenetrable to sperm. This, incidentally, is the main way the progestogen-only pill, known also as the mini-pill, works. It creates the type of cervical secretion that forms a plug and prevents sperm moving out of the vagina. It is often recommended to older women because it is an effective method and has fewer side-effects than the combined pill. But it can cause problems for some women who hope to have children when they come off it. They can be ovulating beautifully but have no fertile mucus for several months before a normal cervical secretion pattern is re-established.

At least some of the information we have been running through will be familiar to you, if not from school, then from books on pregnancy or from the charts in doctors' offices. What you will be less likely to know is how to apply these general rules to yourself so that you can understand your own patterns. The time-honoured method – and the method that a GP may recommend when you first seek help in understanding your fertility – is for you (or, if you are a man, for your partner) – to make a chart of your waking temperatures using a special fertility thermometer and special temperature charts. The official term for this is a basal body temperature chart – BBT for short. If you've had a good night's sleep, if you are not using an electric blanket, if you take your readings before you've had a drink, the temperature tends to be lower during the first part of the cycle, and then rise by about 0.2–0.4 degrees centigrade right after ovulation, in other words under the effect of progesterone. The temperature falls again just before the next period. As you may have noticed, there are a lot of ifs, which is why it is not always easy to interpret a temperature chart. Expert advice is often needed. It is surprising to see how patterns can emerge from what looks at first sight to be a most complicated set of charts. Temperature charts can be useful to reassure women with irregular cycles that they are ovulating. They can also explain why some women are sub-fertile because, if the length of the luteal phase – i.e. the number of days between the temperature rise and the onset of the next period – is very short, this suggests that the empty follicle on the ovary that produces progesterone is failing to produce enough to sustain a pregnancy. If this problem has been identified, then treatment can be given.

Another important pattern to observe is the normal cyclical

changes in cervical secretion. These are harder to understand but it is worth making the effort, as they will reveal far more to you about your cycle than BBT charts. Every woman has a different pattern of secretion. The general rule is that following the end of a period, there is a feeling of dryness at the entrance of the vagina. There is little or no cervical secretion and any in evidence is thick, sticky and white. Some women notice the difference in sensation at the vaginal opening when they walk. As ovulation approaches, the cervical secretions become transparent, thin, stringy and profuse, and she may notice a sensation of lubrication at the vaginal entrance. This is fertile secretion. After ovulation, the cervical secretion returns to the infertile pattern, in other words, becomes thick, sticky and white. In addition to noting the visual differences in cervical secretions, you can also measure its relative stretchiness. This is called the Spinnbarkeit test. Observation of cervical secretion is the best way of predicting ovulation is about to occur. It is often used by couples planning a pregnancy who have intercourse when the fertile mucus is present. The temperature shift occurs *after* ovulation and so only helps to confirm that ovulation has occurred.

Also noteworthy are the changes in the cervix. There are subtle changes which gradually occur in the cervix that a woman can learn to detect if she wishes. They can give a good indication of how her reproductive system is functioning. Women who use IUDs or the diaphragm will have already received some instruction in this area. If you do start to check your cervix, it is important to do so at the same time each day and also in the same position – for example, with a leg raised on a chair, or squatting. The changes you will be looking for will be in the position, shape, and feel of the cervix – whether it is high or low in the vagina, whether it is tilted or not, whether it feels soft or firm to the touch and whether it is slightly open or closed. You will notice that the signs are different during the fertile time compared to early and late in the cycle during the infertile time. As a general rule, a long, low, tilted, firm, dry cervix indicates the infertile time, while a high, short, straight, soft, open, wet cervix indicates the fertile time.

Monitoring cervical secretions and keeping track of changes in the cervix are the main means by which a woman can connect her general knowledge of fertility with her understanding of the way her own reproductive system works. Instruction in this area is usually called fertility awareness. What is the point of fertility awareness? It puts you in charge. Instead of trying to control your body, you can – by getting to know its patterns and idiosyncrasies better – learn how to manage it according to your needs and desires. If you want a baby quickly, you follow one course of action. If you don't want a baby right away, but would not think it the end of the world if one appeared, you follow a different course of action. And if you never ever want another child, you can use the same information base to make sure you never do.

Fertility awareness gives a woman a secure perspective from which to plan her children. Whichever method of family planning she chooses to use, she will understand the implications of misusing the method more clearly. She will also be able to make adjustments. While some women use fertility awareness as their only method of family planning, many other women (particularly women who want more children eventually) chose to use fertility awareness alongside a barrier method. In other words, they use condoms and/or diaphragms in association with a spermicide only during their fertile phase, thus allowing themselves rubber- and chemical-free intercourse during the infertile phase. We would like to emphasise that modern fertility-awareness disciples all want to remove the term 'rhythm method', which is often used as a euphemism for wishful thinking and so has fallen into disrepute.

But before we move on to the subject of contraception, we'd also like to point out that fertility awareness is more than just a tool. It's a different way of *looking* at fertility. It's empirical, in that it takes as its starting point the actual processes of reproduction. It is, in other words, in tune with nature. Our traditional, cultural understanding of fertility is *not* always in tune with nature. We like to see the man and his seed active and daring and abroad, and the woman passively brooding over her tiny, immobile egg. This scenario has little basis in physiological fact, as Mary Ellmann stated so wittily.

> 'An immobility is attributed to the entire female constitution by analogy with the supposed immobility of the ovum. This

> imaginative vision of the ovum, like a pop art fried-egg-on-a-plate, is dependent of course upon a happy physiological vagueness. In actuality, each month the ovum undertakes an extraordinary expedition from the ovary through the fallopian tubes to the uterus, an unseen equivalent of going down the Mississippi on a raft or over Niagara Falls in a barrel. Ordinarily too, the ovum travels singly, like Lewis or Clark, in the kind of existential loneliness which Norman Mailer usually admires. One might say that the activity of ova involves a daring and independence absent, in fact, from the activity of spermatozoa, which move in jostling masses, swarming out on signal like a crowd of commuters from the 5:15.'[4]

Which reminds us of the last point we'd like to make about fertility awareness. Yes, and you'd almost forgotten about them too, hadn't you? Those men, or rather those hundreds of millions of sperm, those commuters without whose assistance not even the most perfect female reproductive system could produce children. Sperm might begin their journey in an undignified way, but the odds against their survival, let alone success, make even life expectancy figures for World War I trench warfare look benign. Many of the original one hundred to three hundred million spermatozoa spill out of the vagina. Most remain in the cervical secretion, with only one in a thousand making it through the cervix. Many of these survivors will be digested by cells in the lining of the uterus. Under two hundred will make it to the egg. Several spermatozoa may penetrate the ovum's outer lining, but only one, you will remember, will actually succeed in fusing with the egg. That's assuming, of course, that there's an egg waiting in the fallopian tube. As we have pointed out, this will not usually be the case. The odds against an individual sperm or, for that matter, an individual egg, ever taking part in a successful conception are so great as to be almost incalculable. From the point of view of its two essential components, birth really does begin to look like a miracle.

For anyone who has ever 'taken chances' and lived to see surprise results, the picture looks altogether different. This brings us to our next subject: how to manage our fertility without inadvertently destroying the fragile processes we have been describing in this chapter.

CHAPTER SIXTEEN

FERTILITY CONTROL: THE CHOICES ON OFFER

As we have pointed out already, originally the main purpose of sex education was fertility control – to teach young people about contraceptives so that they would be able to make the usual mistakes of youth without having to suffer the consequences of early, unplanned pregnancy. The advent of the HIV virus has shifted the focus: if early sexual activity and/or promiscuity was coming to be seen as inadvisable but impossible to prohibit, there is increasing interest today in personal and social education which encourages young people to be able to be say 'no' or at least 'not yet'. Underlying both the permissive- and the epidemic-inspired approaches, is the assumption that sexual feelings and procreative urges lead, if unchecked, to tragically high birth rates and disease, and so must be subjected to vigorous control. Where the answer 'no' is not a likelihood, contraceptives provide the means whereby this control becomes possible.

Isn't that as it should be? What could possibly be wrong with teaching sexually active young people how to exercise what the experts call 'contraceptive vigilance'? The problem as we see it is that the information is presented without regard for context. There is little effort to present fertility as a positive and manageable force – or to give a clear idea how the various forms of contraception act on the reproductive system. If you teach people how to use contraceptives without also telling them how and why they work and what processes they are interrupting; if you teach pregnancy avoidance without first giving people a clear and friendly understanding of their reproductive systems, then you are inadvertently encouraging your students to think about reproduction as a dangerous and hardly controllable force, and setting the scene for compulsive contraceptive 'abuse' – in other words, phases of 'contraceptive vigilance' followed by shameful and spectacular lapses. These lapses are often compounded by people's feelings about authoritarian figures. Many young people are irritated by good advice they get first from parents and later from teachers and other experts. They complain about being told over and over to remain on the straight and narrow path of responsible living and say this does not allow them the space and/or time to discover their own way. There is a need to offer young people time, both in schools and at family planning clinics, to explore how they feel about their sexuality, how they communicate their feelings to others, what they feel ambivalent about, why they might choose to take risks, and whether these risks are calculated or random.

The choice of which method to use is not only based on what you have been taught, but also on how you feel about yourself sexually. How are you going to communicate your chosen method to your partner? Some methods need more co-operation than others.

Another problem, and the one we'll be trying to remedy here, is that because your object when choosing to use contraception is to prevent pregnancy, you will be, at best, only hypothetically interested in the effects the contraceptive might have on your long-term fertility. If the person giving you the information, or, for that matter, the doctor who prescribes the actual device, shares your narrow objectives, then you are not likely to get the full advice you deserve.

These are the pitfalls of what we call the 'contraceptive mentality'. We would like to encourage people instead to look at contraception in the wider context of fertility control. In other words, we would like to see young people getting a full understanding of sexuality and fertility in general and their patterns in particular before their teachers and doctors start working on their emotions and behaviour to produce a desired outcome. The message ought to be: this is your body, this is what it can do, and this is why. You're in charge. You don't have to do what other people tell you to do. Your parents

Fertility Control: the Choices on Offer

might want you to keep your virginity until you're married, your teachers might want you to use contraception so that you don't have to interrupt your studies, your boyfriend might want to have sex without taking any responsibility for contraception, but none of them can make you do what you feel is not right. You're the one to decide if you want five children before you're eighteen, or £50,000 in the bank and fifteen years of full-time work under your belt before you even think of trying for your first. Many people shy away from such tactics, out of fear that they will only encourage immature and socially irresponsible people to become more so, but we believe that the only way to make people truly responsible about their fertility is by teaching them first that it is a power they can be proud of, that they can enjoy exercising, that needs looking after, that is finite and that can be largely under their control.

The first step, if you are to consider contraception in the broader context of fertility control, is to be able to visualise the place of intervention for each contraceptive method and device. In this way we can see that – beginning with the woman – the combined pill shuts off the ovaries, while sterilisation cuts or closes the fallopian tubes. The IUD acts on the lining of the uterus and by impeding sperm from reaching the egg; the diaphragm or female condom or sponge will form a barrier between the penis and the cervix; spermicides work in the vagina, and the progestogen-only pill affects the cervical secretions, or mucus plug. In men, a vasectomy cuts the vas deferens, the tube that transports semen from the testes to the penis, while the condom contains sperm after they have been ejaculated, and withdrawal, or coitus interruptus, is the ejaculation of sperm outside the vagina.

In considering each method separately, it is important to know how it works in theory, how it is used, what effect it is known to have on users' long-term health and fertility, how effective it is and what its practical benefits and drawbacks are. Good family planning already covers all of these areas. If it is falling on deaf ears, it is often because the contraception seeker lacks a solid grounding in fertility. But it is also due to the way in which the information is framed. Few women know to ask, if they have been told that studies indicate a particular device is safe, where and when these studies were conducted, and by whom, and if there are important areas in which studies have yet to be done. They may also get statistical information about positive and negative outcomes, which can be as insidious and nightmarish as ill-defined reports of fluctuating fertility rates, especially if they have no clear visual understanding of how the contraceptive will be acting on their own bodies. And as for the drawbacks of a contraceptive device, they will usually receive some practical information about what it's like to use, and the ways in which previous users have found it annoying, but the effectiveness of a particular device will be represented by two figures, the method-failure rate and the user-failure rate. We are not terribly fond of this last term, as it implies that pregnancy happens to contraceptive users as a result of disobedience, ignorance, wanton carelessness or moral weakness. We think it would be better if people talked instead about (a) the likelihood of a device or method working if you follow the doctor's and the manufacturer's instructions and (b) the reasons you might decide not to use it as instructed, and the likelihood of your making this decision. If effectiveness were more clearly linked to motivation, it would quickly become clear, for example, that a woman who has mixed feelings about a child is far more likely to become pregnant if she uses a method like the pill, which must be taken regularly, or a device like the diaphragm, which she will sometimes be having to interrupt love-making in order to put in – and that she might want a device that works without her assistance like the IUD. Likewise, it would also be clear to a woman who was highly motivated to avoid pregnancy that she stands a chance of doing well even with methods that require willpower. The reputation of a device will also be important. To quote Toni Belfield, Head of Information and Research at the Family Planning Association in London: 'Choice, it seems, is not always based on rational or objective information – the fact that a friend has had a terrible time with the pill or an IUD will have much more influence than any amount of statistics which show this to be unlikely – bad news is always remembered!'[1]

Fertility Control: the Choices on Offer

We will not always be able to follow our own advice as we run through the basic facts about the leading contraceptive devices and gynaecological procedures, because some of the information we would like simply does not exist – or else it is expressed in the terms we find unacceptable for the reasons outlined above. We had problems with some of the accepted terminology – there is, we feel, a worrying tendency to cover up moral problems with euphemisms. One example is the new term 'pre-embryo', which describes a fertilised egg up to day fourteen, which is the time that neural tissue is first visible. The term exists simply to draw a line for researchers. You can do research on pre-embryos, but not on embryos. What happens if Parliament decides to draw this arbitrary line later, at twenty-one days, or twenty-eight days?

We also feel uneasy about the statistical information available on fertility. We rarely found two sources quoting the same figures. This is because studies differ in their results and results are constantly being updated. When in doubt, we tended to go for the more conservative estimate, or else provide an upper as well as a lower figure. As far as our sources went, the ones we ended up trusting most when in doubt were John Guillebaud and Julia Mosse. We recommend both their books to anyone seeking more detailed information than we provide here. But before we continue, we would like to suggest the following questions for all fertility statistics and studies you hear about, both in and outside this book:

Who did it? Was the research done in a major centre? Was the research done by someone whose reputation you know?
Where was it reported? Usually reports emerge from published papers. Have you heard of the journal? A peer-reviewed paper in a well-known journal is usually reliable. A report from a meeting is far less reliable. The 'Shock . . . Horror . . . Breakthrough' reports from the popular press often cause needless anxiety.
Does it make sense? Does it make simple biological sense? Is your credulity strained? If the theory looks daft it probably is. Trust your common sense!
What about numbers? Is it a one-off case report? How many

individuals were involved in the study? How long did the study last? Is it statistically valid? The larger the number the more likely it is that the observation will be correct in its own context – but not necessarily in the cause/effect manner in which it is being presented.

There may be no all round 'perfect' method of family planning, but there usually is a 'good enough' method for your way of life at a particular time. To find it, all you have to do is ask yourself constructive rather than doubt-exacerbating questions. In other words, instead of asking, 'What risks and discomforts am I willing to endure?' better to ask, 'What kind of protection do I most need right now? – A method that preserves me from my own ambivalence? A method that safeguards my future fertility? Or one that allows me to make up my mind on the night of intercourse?'

Remember: risk-taking is not always reckless. It can also be calculated and a means to an end. There is also the question of degree. Most of the statistical risks of pregnancy we will be discussing here are tiny, at least compared to the likelihood of pregnancy for sexually active fertile couples who forgo contraception altogether. We will now review the choices currently on offer for fertility control. Although we have mentioned the main side- effects of each method it is only a very small minority who will ever experience them.

The Combined Oral Contraceptive Pill

How it works: The combined oral contraceptive pill contains a combination of the hormones oestrogen and progestogen. The oestrogen prevents ovulation by maintaining hormonal levels in such a way that the follicles on the ovaries do not ripen and so eggs are not released. The progestogen will make the cervical secretions thick and sticky and impenetrable to sperm.

How it is used: The user must take one pill a day for twenty-one days and then stop for seven days, when a withdrawal bleed (not a period, and usually lighter than a period) will occur due to decreased levels of hormones. (There are some brands of pill that contain twenty-eight pills, the last seven being pills which contain no hormones so that the less methodical user knows to take a pill every day.) A leaflet explaining about the combined pill is also essential including clear instructions about what to do if you miss a pill, if you are ill or if you take medication. It is essential to have regular check-ups usually every six months.

Effectiveness: It is one of the most reliable methods if used correctly. It requires the user to acknowledge her fertility and sexual intentions on a daily basis. Method-failure accounts for pregnancies in 0.2 per hundred women taking the pill for a year. Because many women forget to take their tablets, or else take them too late, or in conjunction with certain antibiotics without using other protection for intercourse, the general failure rate is one per hundred women taking the pill for a year.[2] With less careful use up to seven women in a hundred will get pregnant in one year. The combined pill is a potential money-spinner for drug companies, and so very well-advertised and promoted, often with statistics that family planning clinics are inclined to question.

Suitability: The pill is suitable for most women unless they have been identified as having one of the following contra-indications: past history of previous blood clots, heart disease or angina, raised blood lipids (fats), severe high blood pressure, stroke or focal migraine, diabetes any previous severe liver disease and any cancer which may be dependent on hormones such as cancer of the breast or endometrium. You should not take it if you think you might be pregnant or are experiencing any abnormal vaginal bleeding. Women who are heavy smokers or are very overweight should be counselled carefully, as should those with a strong family history of heart disease.

Risks and benefits: Although the pills on the market today contain lower doses of hormones than their antecedents and are therefore safer, the pill has been linked to many health problems. Some users complain that it affects their mood and even libido and causes them to gain weight, while for women who began using the pill when very young there is some evidence that there is possibly a small increased risk of breast cancer, and there may be a slightly increased risk of cancer of the cervix. Nowadays many women are encouraged to use a barrier method, e.g. a condom, as well as the pill to protect against sexually transmitted diseases (STDs), especially now because of the anxiety about the HIV virus. This combination of pill plus condom is often called the Double Dutch method. The combined pill decreases the risk of cancer of the endometrium (uterine lining) and cancer of the ovary. At present, research seems to indicate that the overall risk of cancer is not greater than for the general population. The pill can contribute to the risk of thrombo-embolism (blood clots forming in veins, especially those in the legs) and other blood vessel diseases including high blood pressure. Smokers over thirty-five years of age run a significantly higher risk of coronary heart disease if they use the pill, so it is no longer recommended for these women.

It is not clear what effect the combined pill has on long-term fertility – there is room for more studies in this area – but it is generally agreed that not all women resume ovulating within six to eight weeks after coming off the pill. Sometimes this will be blamed on the pill when other factors – such as increased age or previous abnormal cycles – might be to blame. According to John Guillebaud, previously fertile women who have come off the pill are just as likely as fertile non pill-users to have had their next child within thirty months, but he does concede that former pill-users seem to take three to twelve months longer than non-users to conceive, especially if the woman concerned has never conceived before and/or is over the age of thirty.[3]

Many women who are on the pill do not seem to have been told this. It is a fact that may not be of importance to someone in her early thirties: even if she wants several children, she has quite a few years to play with – but if a woman plans to come off the pill in her late thirties, with just enough time to produce two children before she turns forty, she will need to know that there is a possibility she'll have to wait before conceiving.

Also vulnerable are girls who went on the pill when their cycles were irregular and anovulatory. This is ironic, as a classic reason for doctors putting such girls on the pill is to 'make their periods regular'. As John Guillebaud states, 'It is illogical for the combined pill to be used to simply "regularise" infrequent irregular periods. After all, "Pill periods" are entirely artificial.'[4] If, however, a woman can establish that she is not ovulating even after coming off the combined pill, she can kick-start her ovaries by taking drugs that stimulate the ovaries such as Clomiphene or Pergonal. These types of drugs are the ones that have made triplets, quads, and quins more common in the past, but they are better administered today than they were, and so the chance of multiple pregnancy is far less common.

As there is continuing research about the long-term effects of the pill, and as results are often contradictory, confusing, and hard to apply to the individual case, we reproduce here the set of questions that John Guillebaud recommends a woman to ask when confronted with data from a new study:

(1) How strong is the evidence? Has it been consistently shown by more than one group of researchers? And/or is there a reason for expecting the effect, such as a known change in body chemistry?
(2) How important is the condition being caused, worsened, or improved?
(3) How large is the effect of the pill? (How many times more or less common is the condition in pill-users?)
(4) How common is the condition anyway?[5]

One must also bear in mind that the pills used in the past were given at higher doses than present-day pills and hence the side-effects were more marked. The type of progestogen has also been changed.
Misuse of the method: If a woman forgets to take the pill for longer than twelve hours from the time she usually takes her tablet, the suppressive effect of the pill on the follicles on the ovaries will gradually reduce, and the body's natural hormones may cause a follicle on one of the ovaries to rupture and release an egg. The only way of stopping the sperm from reaching the egg is either to avoid intercourse or to use a combined barrier method such as a condom and spermicidal for the next seven days. If she has either diarrhoea, vomiting or is on a course of certain antibiotics, the pill may not be absorbed in the normal way and the above scenario might occur. In this instance, she should use a barrier method for the duration of the illness or course of antibiotics and for the next seven days.

The Progestogen-Only Pill

How it works: The progestogen-only pill, or mini-pill as it used to be called, maintains a constant level of the hormone progestogen which maintains a mucus plug within the cervix throughout the cycle. Its main action is like that of a barrier method. To quote John Guillebaud: 'Consider the progestogen-only pill as a barrier method that is taken by mouth.'[6] Even if you're ovulating, no sperm are supposed to be able to get through it. If some do and an egg is fertilised, the progestogen will also have affected the uterine lining and so prevent implantation. The progestogen-only pill prevents ovulation in twenty per cent of women. About forty per cent ovulate occasionally and forty per cent continue to ovulate normally.

How it is used: A pill is taken every day, including during the periods, i.e. 365 days of the year. It is very important to take the pill at the same time of day. The mucus is at its thickest about four to five hours after taking the pill. It is important to have regular check-ups every six months.

Effectiveness: If taken regularly the failure rate is 0.3 to 4 per hundred women taking the pill for a year.[7] It is more effective in thin women compared to women over seventy kilos. It is also more effective in women over thirty-five years, as are all other methods.

Suitability: The pill is especially suitable for breast-feeding women, because the amount of progestogen (see Glossary) passing to the baby via the milk is minimal. Older women and women who have had problems with the combined pill linked to oestrogen and women who continue to smoke and are over the age of thirty-five are also frequently prescribed it. The relative contra-indications are: a past history of ectopic pregnancy, previous blood clots, heart disease or angina, raised blood lipids (fats), severe high blood pressure, stroke or focal migraine, any previous severe liver disease and any cancer which may be dependent on hormones such as cancer of the breast or endometrium. You should not take it if you think you might be pregnant, or are experiencing any abnormal vaginal bleeding. Women who are heavy smokers or are very overweight should be counselled carefully before using this type of contraception.

Risks and benefits: The progestogen-only pill causes an irregular bleeding pattern in about forty per cent of users, and at least twenty per cent have no periods at all. This may cause unnecessary anxiety about a pregnancy, which makes it unacceptable to some women. Some users complain that it causes headaches, affects their mood and libido and causes them to gain weight. Overall these side-effects are much less frequent than with the combined pill. It is the safer of the two methods, which is why it is so often prescribed to older women who have been advised not to use the combined pill. However, it is not as effective a method as the combined oral contraceptive, largely because it does not work unless the user takes a pill at the same time every day. There may be a very slightly increased risk of ectopic pregnancies (one per thousand women on the pill every year),[8] which may affect the future fertility of a woman who has not completed her family. It is therefore important she is counselled about this. There is generally less disruption to the cycle after coming off the progestogen-only pill but some women may experience disruption to the mucus pattern.

Misuse of the method: This pill is not for the forgetful type. If you do forget to take the progestogen-only pill and are more than three hours late, the mucus may change from the thick plug into fertile mucus which the sperm can swim through. As we have already said, only twenty per cent of women on this type of pill never ovulate, so there might be an egg ready for fertilisation. It is therefore very important to use a combined barrier method such as condoms and spermicidals for the next seven days and continue to take your pill. If you have either vomiting or severe diarrhoea, the pill may not be absorbed in the normal way and the above scenario might happen. You should therefore use a barrier method carefully for the duration of the illness, plus another seven days.

Injectable Progestogen
How it works: A high dose of a Progestogen is injected into a muscle.

It steadily releases progestogen into the circulation at a higher level than the progestogen-only pill. It prevents ovulation and also forms a hostile mucus plug.

How it is used: The injection must be given in the first five days of the cycle, usually during a period. It is essential to have regular check-ups. There are two preparations used at present: Depo-Provera, which must be injected every twelve weeks, and is far more widely used, and Norethisterone Oenanthate, which must be injected every eight weeks and is only licensed for short-term use, for example, by the partners of men being sterilised. WHO is developing a once-a-month injectable, which may cause less menstrual disruption. As with other Progestogen-only preparations it is not uncommon for women to experience irregular frequent bleeding in the first two months of using Depo-Provera but this usually settles down. Often periods become less frequent or cease altogether. In Britain it is recommended that a doctor should authorise an injection of Depo-Provera only after the patient has read and understood an official leaflet.

Effectiveness: This is an extremely effective method, with 0–1 failures per hundred women using the method for a year, because it does not depend on a woman's daily motivation to work.

Suitability: This method is suitable for the forgetful woman, and is frequently offered by family planning clinics to women who are disorganised in their family planning (i.e. who have had many abortions), and who have already got several children.

It is not ideal for a woman who is planning a family because she should expect to wait at least a year before conceiving after she has had her last injection.

Risks and benefits: Although it has the advantage of lasting for three months, the main disadvantage is that injections cannot be reversed so any side-effects, such as no periods, excessive bleeding, headaches, mood changes, lack of libido and problem weight-gain may persist for three months. Injectable contraceptives got a bad name in the sixties and seventies because of the irresponsible licensing and international misuse of Depo-Provera. The advantages are that it is effective in preventing pregnancy, and shown by studies to be protective against pelvic inflammatory disease.

Misuse of the method: This is not a method that can be misused as long as the patient has her injections regularly.

Norplant[32]

How it works: Norplant is a progestogen implant designed to provide contraception for five years. It consists of six flexible sealed silastic tubes (roughly 34 mm long) containing slow release progestogen. The tubes are inserted in a fan-shaped pattern in the upper inner part of the left arm in the right-handed woman.

It has to be inserted by a trained health professional using a local anaesthetic. The procedure takes about fifteen minutes. Removal, which can be complicated by fibrous tissue formation, usually takes about thirty minutes. (Biodegradable implants are being developed.) Women given Norplant should be entered on a register. This will ensure that they can be contacted if there emerge any unexpected side-effects. It will also mean that they can be reminded that the device needs to be removed when the five years are up.

Effectiveness: Studies have shown less than one pregnancy per hundred women years. However, the risk of pregnancy in heavier women (i.e. over 70 kilos) is up to 7.6 per hundred women years. There is no user-failure risk with Norplant. If pregnancy does occur, it is important to check whether it is ectopic, as there is a high incidence of this complication occurring amongst the tiny fraction of Norplant users who conceive.[33]

Suitability: Although Norplant has been heralded as a useful way of preventing teenage pregnancy, it has been licensed in the UK for women aged 18–40. It is being targeted at women who have had difficulty with contraceptive methods that require high motivation. It would also benefit any woman who is reasonably sure she does not want children for at least five years. *All* women should have counselling prior to insertion.

Risks and Benefits: The system has a high incidence of side-effects. Some are related to the progestogen. These include irregular bleeding [34,35] (in 50–80 per cent of users) and headaches (in 50–80 per cent) and the other side-effects associated with the progestogen-only pill. Side-effects associated with the Norplant tubes include skin irritation, occasional infection, increased pigmentation and fibrous tissue build-up. They are palpable under the skin and may be visible when the arm is extended. Due to these problems the mean continuation time is only 3.5 years.[34]

The advantage of Norplant over the progestogen injection is that it can be removed if there are side-effects. However as this is an expensive method (£179 for the device, plus the costs for counselling, follow-up, insertion and removal), there is a debate about how to make it cost-effective and obviously women will be encouraged to use it for longer periods rather than shorter ones.

Future Developments: Coming at some point is the vaginal ring, which will release either spermicide or hormones, and will be able to remain in place for between one and three months. Trials have shown that women find this method very convenient.[10] The vaginal ring called Femring, which releases a low dose of progestogen over ninety days, is simple to use and easily reversible. It has side-effects similar to those associated with the progestogen-only pill but the bleeding pattern is more erratic and there are also specific side-effects related to the ring such as vaginal irritation and discharge. The levels of progestogen are lower than those of the implant and the failure rate is about three pregnancies per hundred women using the method for a year. A ring containing oestrogen and progestogen is also being developed. Other ways of delivering progestogen under consideration are an IUD containing progestogen, and an intra-cervical device that is inserted into the cervix and contains progestogen or a spermicidal.[11] The former is now completing trials in the UK. Vaccination against pregnancy is another idea in long-term development.

The Female Barrier Methods

How they work: The models of choice today are of three types: the diaphragm, the vault cap and the cervical cap.[12] They are inserted into the vagina in such a way as to prevent the penis being in direct contact with the cervix during intercourse. To be effective, they must be used in conjunction with a spermicidal cream, gel, foam, film or pessary. These create a contraceptive layer that keeps any sperm which may leak around the cap from passing through the cervix. The cervix usually is situated at the back of the upper wall of the vagina. The diaphragm lies covering the cervix along the entire upper wall of the vagina. It is the most common type of diaphragm used, and comes in a variety of sizes. The vault and vimule caps lie covering the cervix at the upper end of the vagina. The vault cap is ideal for a short, wide cervix and for a woman having difficulty with the diaphragms staying in place due to lax muscles. The vimule combines the characteristics of the vault and cervical caps and is ideal for a woman with an irregular or cone shaped cervix. The cervical cap fits directly over the cervix and is only suitable for a woman with a long healthy cervix which is not pointing backwards.

How they are used: Whatever type of cap is used, all types of caps and diaphragms must be fitted carefully, and a woman must be given time to learn to use it in an unhurried atmosphere (a sense of humour is very helpful), so that she is sure she knows how to check she has covered the cervix. Instruction about how to use the spermicide must be clearly explained and she must also be given written instructions. The protection from the initial application of spermicidal cream or gel lasts for about three hours and/or one act of intercourse. For protection in the event of another act of intercourse, it is necessary to use more spermicide – non-oil based gel or cream with an applicator, or a pessary. Cervical caps can remain in place for no longer than thirty hours, with a need for extra spermicide in the event of a second or subsequent act of intercourse. You must keep all these devices in place for at least six hours after intercourse.

Effectiveness: Recent studies have shown that older users with completed families who had used the diaphragm for more than four years had a 0.7 failure rate, while other studies for less specific groups put the failure rate as high as fifteen per hundred women using the cap for a year.

Suitability: Although it is free of any serious health hazards and once learnt is easy to use, only two per cent of women in this country use the diaphragm. This may be because it is a method that requires a matter-of-fact attitude to bodily processes: many people – even people who have been through the indignities of childbirth – are squeamish about putting their hand 'in there'. Even those who are comfortable with their bodies may find compliance with the instructions irksome and impractical. Getting out of bed halfway through lovemaking to go into a bathroom to put in a diaphragm has a way of putting a damper on things.

Risks and benefits: The diaphragm and the cap are among the safest contraceptives available. The diaphragm does predispose some women to urinary infections, but it (or the spermicides) provide increased protection against pelvic inflammatory disease (PID), cervical cancer, and AIDS. There have been studies indicating that spermicides in use at the time of conception are linked with birth defects, but their findings have been seriously questioned. Although women with certain shapes of vagina have problems with the cap being dislodged during intercourse in certain positions (in the US, ten to twenty-five per cent of all women asking for the cap were not able to be fitted), the diaphragm is quite reliable *if* you follow instructions.

Misuse of the method: Obviously, this method requires motivation. It is not uncommon for a woman to choose not to use it at the actual time of intercourse and in the heat of the moment, for whatever reason. This may well explain the higher failure rate figure. Putting it in every night 'just in case' is the solution that many women now find most acceptable. Traditionally, a prepared woman has been seen as 'forward', but all that is changing, and wearing a diaphragm and carrying condoms in your handbag (or wearing them as earrings) is seen as 'responsible'. Putting it in before you go out for an evening with someone you don't know very well may mean admitting to yourself, and possibly even to him, that you're available, but so what?

It is possible to miss the cervix altogether and put in the diaphragm without covering it, because the cervix, as we have already explained, moves up and down the vagina during a typical cycle. In fact, the cervix is at the *highest* position at the most fertile time of the cycle, which will be the time it is most difficult for a woman to check it, and hence a time when she is most likely to make mistakes. If she inserts the cap incorrectly, there will be nothing to stop the sperm travelling up through the cervix, especially if there is not enough spermicide present. This information ought to be routinely given to women who are fitted with a diaphragm.

Other female barrier methods: Other barrier methods include spermicides used on their own. These are generally effective only about two-thirds of the time, and so are not recommended by professionals in this country. The contraceptive sponge is available over the counter. It is easy to put in but is often inserted incorrectly. It works for twenty-four hours at a time and should always remain in place for six hours after intercourse. The failure rate is as high as 24.5 per cent and so it is only recommended to women who appreciate its convenience and who are spacing children rather than seeking to avoid pregnancy altogether. The female condom is a loose strong polyurethane tube with a ring at the top and the bottom. The upper ring is designed to cover the cervix, while the lower ring lies outside the vagina. It is said to be as easy to use as a male condom, but it has not been tested enough yet for us to know just how effective it is or how popular it will prove to be. Its potential in the prevention of HIV is a significant issue. Other barrier methods being developed are a custom-made cervical cap and a disposable diaphragm.

The Male Barrier Method

How it works: The condom is made of high-standard latex, sometimes with a teat at the end to collect the sperm. It is usually coated with a lubricant which often also contains a spermicide. There are all sorts of different types on offer: ribbed condoms, coloured condoms, condoms made of reinforced rubber for anal intercourse. There are 'non-allergenic' condoms for those who develop an allergy to rubber or to the spermicidal.

How it is used: The condom is fitted over the erect penis and, if used correctly, it will prevent sperm from entering the vagina. It is recommended that the woman also uses a spermicidal in case of condom failure.

Effectiveness: It is effective if used with care, with a pregnancy rate of two to fifteen per hundred couples using the method for a year.

Suitability: There are no medical risks. Success depends very much on motivation of the couple.

Risks and benefits: The condom is the only form of contraception for which the man takes responsibility other than sterilisation. It protects the couple from the HIV virus and other diseases as well as preventing pregnancy – if it doesn't burst or slip off or get punctured by fingernails. Although quality control is stringent in the UK, and although the official bursting rate is only 1.4 per hundred couple-years, many people do complain about such mishaps. One result of its recent comeback as a result of the AIDS epidemic is that accidental pregnancy due to defective condoms is on the increase, but figures may be misleading, as it is also a convenient and respectable excuse which can be used to explain why you got pregnant when you are seeking an abortion. Some women come off the pill if the couple have decided they will use the condom anyway because of HIV, and this may be another reason.

Misuse of the method: The most common reason for condom failure is inconsistent or improper use. Maximum effectiveness is achieved when the following rules are observed: (1) Use a condom every time. (2) Avoid any damage to the condom when opening the foil pack. (3) Unroll the condom over the erect penis before any genital contact, pinching the teat or plain end to expel air. (4) After intercourse, withdraw the penis before it becomes too soft, holding the base of the condom during withdrawal and taking care not to spill any semen. (5) Use only kite-marked condoms, and each condom only once. (6) Do *not* use Vaseline or other oil-based lubricant on the condom as it will dissolve the condom. If additional lubrication is desired, use K-Y jelly or spermicidal jelly.[13]

Intra-Uterine Contraception

How it works: The intra-uterine device or IUD is a small device, often but not always T-shaped, made of plastic with copper wound round it. It is placed in the uterine cavity, where it causes an adverse environment for the sperm and the egg. The copper impedes the motility of the sperm. It also affects the lining of the uterus. So now it seems that it does actually prevent fertilisation at least some of the time, rather than implantation.

How it is used: The IUD must be inserted by a trained doctor, often at the end of a period so one can be sure the woman is not pregnant. While it is important to remain wary of the risks, it is also possible for the user to stay one step ahead of the game by checking for the thread once a month. If you can't feel the thread, this could mean the IUD has slipped or been involuntarily expelled from the uterus, and obviously, the sooner you know there is a problem, the better. If you don't like doing this check, you can always get a family planning doctor or nurse to check it for you.

Effectiveness: It has an overall 0.3–2 per cent failure rate per hundred women using this method for one year.

Suitability: Seven per cent of women between eighteen and forty-four in this country depend on the IUD for birth control, with the device's popularity increasing with the user's age. Because of the risk of infection, which can affect the fallopian tubes and therefore fertility, the IUD is not encouraged in young childless women. (It is also harder to insert in childless women.) But it is a popular and reliable enough method for women who have had all the children they want and are not quite ready for the final solution, that is sterilisation.

Risks and benefits: Most problems occur soon after the IUD has been fitted. During the first month of use, the chances of an infection which if not treated properly may result in pelvic inflammatory disease (or PID) are four times what they are for a woman not using contraception. If a woman experiences persistent low abdominal pain after an IUD is inserted, it is important she seeks medical advice early, so that infection is treated quickly and any damage to the fallopian tubes is minimised. By four months, the risk of PID is no different than that faced by the general population, except for women who have been exposed to sexually transmitted diseases. The device can also be involuntarily expelled. This is estimated to happen to between one and fifteen per cent of all users. It usually happens during the first three months and is more likely to happen if the woman is young, has never been pregnant or has just had an abortion or delivered a baby. The skill of the fitter is also a factor. Other risks include a perforated womb or cervix, which 0.6 to 1.2 per cent of users suffer, again largely thanks to bad fitting. Side-effects include increased bleeding and pain, which causes up to twenty per cent of women to discontinue use.

If a woman becomes pregnant with an IUD in place, she will have a three to nine per cent risk of an ectopic pregnancy. If this occurs, it is not only a life-threatening event, but can also affect her fertility afterwards, as she may have to have the affected tube removed. We have been assured that those babies you've all heard about who were born clutching IUDs were holding devices no longer on the market. It is often possible, however, for a doctor to gently remove an IUD after the confirmation of pregnancy: the chance of a miscarriage following this procedure is twenty to thirty per cent, which is lower than if the IUD remains. In the thirty per cent of cases where the ultrasound scan cannot locate the IUD, the chance of a miscarriage becomes fifty-five per cent, or three times the normal rate. Many of these occur in the second trimester – the chances of a miscarriage during this trimester are twenty-five times the normal rate. Prematurity is also more common in IUD pregnancies.

Misuse of the method: If a woman fails to check the thread each month there is a small possibility the device may have either fallen out or moved away from the uterine cavity. If this has happened there will be nothing to prevent a pregnancy occurring.[14]

Natural Family Planning

How it works: Natural family planning depends on accurately defining your fertile time during each cycle. This is done by recording: the temperature on waking patterns, cervical secretion patterns, the changes in the cervix, and other indicators. This type of natural family planning is known as the 'sympto-thermal' or 'multiple index' method. Ultrasound scanning techniques which can detect ovulation have confirmed the accuracy of this method.

How it is used: A woman is taught to avoid intercourse during the fertile time if she doesn't want to get pregnant, and to have intercourse during that time if she does. If she and her partner are avoiding intercourse, they must be counselled carefully about how

Fertility Control: the Choices on Offer

this period of abstinence is going to affect their relationship.

Well-designed charts are essential, as are special fertility thermometers, with a smaller range of temperatures and more widely spaced indices. You need to work with an expert for at least three months and preferably six months before you can really know how to interpret your own patterns, and give due weight to external factors (such as sleep patterns, illness, stress, diet, travel, etc.) that may affect your measurements. The Bioself is a thermometer combined with a computer that bleeps green on 'safe' days. It is becoming more reliable but is expensive. There are several similar devices being developed.

It is impossible to give a full account of the sympto-thermal method here, because so much depends on each individual's pattern. We shall therefore give an overview – and stress again that if you want to use this method you need to learn it from an experienced teacher. The Clubb, Pyper and Knight Oxford Study showed that it took on average four hours of teaching to learn the method fully.[15]

The fertile cervical secretions occur in most women some days after the period has ended and several days before ovulation occurs. Some women with short cycles have fertile mucus immediately after a period. These secretions warn a woman ovulation is approaching and the infertile phase before ovulation has ended. If she does not want to conceive, she learns to avoid intercourse on days there is any mucus – and, for safety's sake, also avoiding intercourse on the following day. (It is best to check this with your teacher.)

The tell-tale rise on the temperature chart does not occur until just after ovulation has occurred. This temperature rise enables a woman to establish the infertile phase after ovulation. Using the two indicators together as well as other signs such as the state of the cervix (which around the time of ovulation is upright, high in the vagina, soft and more open), it is possible to be more accurate about the time of ovulation. The rule is that you can have intercourse without running the risk of conception if you have three consecutive temperature readings that are higher than the previous six, and you have not had any fertile mucus for the last four days.

It takes time to learn the method, and it requires diligent record-keeping, but once you learn it, all you have to do is start taking your temperature around day seven, look out for fertile mucus, and then act according to your current script dictates until there have been three early-morning temperatures higher by 0.2 degrees centigrade than the previous six.

Some women using natural family planning mainly keep track of their cervical secretions. This is called the 'ovulation method' or the 'Billings method', which is generally found to be less reliable than the sympto-thermal method.[16]

Effectiveness: If the couple are motivated and the sympto-thermal method is taught by an experienced teacher, the failure rate is between 1.1 to 3.9 per cent of women using the method for one year. Several recent studies in Europe have confirmed these figures. This failure rate is on a par with barrier methods.

In some studies in the developing world the user failure rates have been unacceptably high at 5 to 15.4 per cent of women using the method for one year. This is thought to be due to less competent teachers.[17]

Suitability: Any couple can learn about natural family planning. It is the one method available that requires and delivers a full fertility awareness that is independent of a desired outcome. The sympto-thermal method has received much support from various cultures and religious groups around the world, and most recently from women interested in the Green movement (as the method is chemical-free). It is designed to work on its own. It is not necessary, and often unhelpful, to have a high level of education if you are trying to use natural family planning.

Motivation is separate from information – in other words, you can use the same charting methods to avoid pregnancy or achieve it. The assumption is that you will want different outcomes at different points in your life. Because it provides such a broad approach to fertility, it is useful to take a course in natural family planning even if you never intend to use it as a method of birth control.

Risks and benefits: It has no side-effects and, if the couple is well-motivated, it is a very effective method. Fertility awareness gives all women an independence based on the knowledge of how their own body works. Rather than thinking of their body as clockwork, they learn to understand, accept, and interpret fluctuations within the norm. They will not panic, therefore, if they see that they are sometimes having anovular cycles or if their luteal (post-ovulation) phase is so short that they could never sustain a pregnancy even if an egg were to be fertilised. Even if women are breast-feeding and not having periods, they will be able to tell when they are about to ovulate by monitoring changes in the cervix and keeping track of their mucus. And, perhaps most important, they learn to anticipate, and communicate, changes in motivation.

The drawbacks to using it are mainly practical. It requires methodical recording and consistent interpretation of the charts. Avoiding intercourse during the fertile time can cause emotional stress for the couple, which, if unresolved, will lead to larger problems. It is very important, therefore, for the issue of abstinence to be addressed and continually re-examined. There may come a time when the couple decides that abstinence is creating more problems than it is solving.

A good source of further reading on this subject is *Fertility: A Comprehensive Guide to Natural Family Planning* by Dr Elizabeth Clubb and Jane Knight.

Misuse of the method: Very often women will try to use the method properly and fail because they have relied on information they got from a book, a TV programme, or a friend. It is one thing to grasp the principles of natural birth control and quite another to apply these principles to your own case. Another prerequisite for natural birth control is a stable life. This is not a method that is well-suited to chaotic routines and emotional upheavals. It is designed for couples, and again, for the method to work properly, both the man and the woman must be motivated, and ideally both should attend the training sessions. Some men don't like natural family planning, as the method puts women in control of the timing of intercourse. Some women find that their husbands refuse to go anywhere near them when they give them the green light, announce that ovulation has definitely occurred, and that sex is now safe. Other men tackle the problem head on by taking charge of all record keeping. One natural family planning teacher told us about an eminent scientist who took control of his wife's charts, insisting that he could read them better than anyone. He then made an elaborate mathematical calculation why it was OK to make love on a night when it was patently obvious that it was not OK. We are happy to report that after his wife became pregnant, he took full responsibility for his error.

Barrier methods and fertility awareness: Many women who have received tuition in natural family planning go on to use barriers during their fertile phase. At this point, it ceases to be natural family planning. Instead it is the barrier method modified by fertility awareness. It is harder for women using this combined method to identify different kinds of cervical secretions, but it is not impossible, especially for the woman who is familiar with her fertility pattern.

Breast-Feeding

This is rarely recommended to an individual as a form of reliable birth control, but lactational amenorrhoea is estimated to be the most effective way of keeping world population levels down. Women who are 'fully' breast-feeding – i.e. not offering their baby any solid or liquid supplements other than water – will usually not ovulate, or have periods. Even when they are supplementing the breast-feeds with food some women do not ovulate for a year or sometimes even two. It has also been shown that breast-feeding women tend to have very short luteal (post-ovulatory) phases, which means that even if an egg becomes fertilised, the pregnancy is unlikely to be sustained long enough for that egg to implant in the wall of the uterus. If you want to have another child, but not right away, breast-feeding might be a suitable form of birth control. Otherwise, it might be a bad idea if used as the only method of family planning.

Women who understand their normal pattern of cervical secretions can use natural family planning successfully while breast-feeding if they are taught by an experienced teacher. It is far less easy to teach a woman who has never learnt fertility awareness before.

Female Sterilisation

How it works: Female sterilisation means having clips, or 'occlusive devices' put on your fallopian tubes, or else having whole sections of the tube cut. The first method is the most recent and most popular.[18] It is estimated that fifteen per cent of women between the ages of sixteen and forty-nine in this country have been sterilised.[19] If you include male sterilisation, twenty-five per cent of couples in this country depend on sterilisation for birth control, and ninety-five million world-wide![20]

How it is done: Female sterilisation is an operation that is carried out under a local anaesthetic or a general anaesthetic which has its own risks. Surgical techniques have been improved over the last ten years and it is usually carried out as a day case. A laparoscope (which is a small telescope) is used in most women and only a small incision is necessary. It is essential to counsel a woman and ideally the couple before carrying out a sterilisation. The couple must understand the small risk of failure. They should have space to discuss both the short-term and long-term implications of the decision. (If a couple is married, it is no longer mandatory to have the husband's signature.)[21]

Effectiveness: The procedure is almost, but not a hundred per cent effective, with the occlusive devices having a slightly higher failure rate – failure meaning, of course, pregnancy.

Suitability: The method is only for couples who are absolutely certain they have completed their family. Although some doctors are over-zealous about recommending sterilisation to women they feel have had enough children, there is a general reluctance to perform sterilisation on women who are under twenty-five years old unless there is a compelling reason such as a severe problem related to pregnancy, and they will usually be advised to think very carefully before making a decision.

Risks and benefits: Although sterilisation involves some pain due to the operation, if all is well the couple have an almost one hundred per cent effective method of contraception which is immediately effective. The woman does not usually need any further medical intervention and there are no important long-term side-effects. Any surgical procedure carries its own risk including the risk of the general anaesthetic, and there are more complications related to female sterilisation than to vasectomy. Although many women express relief following sterilisation, John Guillebaud notes that 'Psychologically though illogically, women may feel no longer so feminine because they cannot have babies.'[22] It is therefore important that counselling is offered.

Reversal of the method: Although only three per cent of sterilised women ask for reversals,[23] 'regret' is reported in about forty per cent of all sterilised women. This seems most likely to happen if the decision was made quickly at a time of crisis, or under pressure from a partner or doctor. There is a greater possibility of reversal if you have clips but, even then, much depends on the skill of the surgeon. The success rates for the best surgeons are as high as eighty per cent, but some people believe that this figure is high because these surgeons have a rigorous selection procedure. Other sources quote a thirty to fifty-five per cent success rate. Just because the fallopian tubes are intact, it does not mean that eggs will be able to move through them in the same way afterwards. Two women in a hundred, conceiving after a reversal, will experience ectopic pregnancies – this is twice the normal risk.

Male Sterilisation or Vasectomy

How it works: Vasectomy is the birth control choice for thirteen per cent of couples in this country, and thirty-three million couples world-wide. It involves interrupting or making a cut in the two tubes, called the vas deferens, that transport sperm from each testicle to the penis. It should have no effect on the man's ability to have erections, orgasms, ejaculations, or sex. The production of seminal fluid continues: it simply contains no sperm.

How it is done: A vasectomy operation is relatively simple. It is carried out as an outpatient procedure and is performed under local anaesthetic. It involves a small incision in the scrotum. The vas deferens on either side is identified and cut and tied. The skin incision is then closed. It is essential that the couple understand that it doesn't work right away for anyone. First you have to get rid of the sperm already in the semen. (This does not have to be through ejaculation: sperm will eventually disintegrate on their own.) Before a man is considered clear in this country, he must have provided two sperm-free semen samples, one ten weeks after the operation, and one after twelve weeks.

Effectiveness: The procedure is almost, but not a hundred per cent effective. Sometimes if the operation is not carried out properly there is a spontaneous reversal. The failure rate is one in a thousand.

Suitability: The method is only suitable for couples who are absolutely certain they have completed their family.

Risks and benefits: The operation sometimes causes bruising and pain, although this is often very slight and brief. Swelling and/or fluid build-up occurs in a few (this too can be easily treated). Any infections that result will usually respond to antibiotics. At present there is conflicting evidence as to whether a vasectomy slightly increases the risk of developing cancer of the prostate gland.

Reversal of the method: In the UK, only one in a thousand men ask for reversals. The odds for a successful reversal have improved with microsurgery: estimates range from thirty-five to ninety-one per cent. It seems that the sooner a reversal is attempted, the likelier it is to succeed. But the presence of sperm in a man's semen does not automatically imply he can father children. Some men manufacture antibodies to their own sperm after a vasectomy. Some studies show that the likelihood of fathering a child after a vasectomy reversal is thirty per cent; other studies claim it is as high as sixty per cent. Some work has been done on a temporary plug for the vas deferens. Another recommended measure is the storage of sperm from men before they are sterilised. This is not available on the NHS.

Emergency Contraception

Emergency contraception exists in the twilight zone between contraception and abortion. While it is true that it may be intervening after a fertilisation, instead of preventing fertilisation in the manner of 'true' contraception, it prevents implantation. The same is possibly true (at least some of the time) of the IUD and the progestogen-only pill. Also, a woman will be seeking emergency contraception not after a confirmed pregnancy, but after an episode of unprotected intercourse. In most cases, therefore, she will not actually be pregnant.

The 'morning-after pill' is a term that is misleading because it is a method which can be used within seventy-two hours of any previous episodes of unprotected intercourse. It consists of four of the stronger combined contraceptive tablets, taken in two doses, twelve hours apart. The pills work because the high dose of oestrogen and progestogen makes the uterine lining build up suddenly and then, as the oestrogen and progestogen levels just as suddenly drop off, so that the tissue cannot be maintained, and a period usually results. A woman may experience nausea or even vomiting. If vomiting occurs within three hours of taking the pills a further dose should be taken immediately. The high dose of oestrogen and progestogen may disrupt periods for a while afterwards. The method is not a hundred per cent effective, although there seem to be no fetal abnormalities in babies born to mothers who attempted the treatment. One thing most people do not know is that an IUD can be inserted up to five days after unprotected intercourse. This will either prevent implantation or the motility of sperm, with about ninety-nine per cent effectiveness. A post-coital IUD is more effective than hormonal methods if there has been unprotected intercourse over a period of days. It is important, though, to be very sure of your dates, because putting an IUD into a pregnant uterus is both illegal and very dangerous.[24]

A recent study in Oxford found that of the 733 women who had abortions, seventy per cent of them could have used emergency contraception, but thirty per cent had never heard of it.

Another much more controversial and not precisely legal method of emergency contraception is menstrual extraction, also known as 'DIY abortion'. This involves sucking out the contents of the uterus at the time a woman is expecting her period, in other words, before she has any evidence that she might be pregnant. If a woman has a symptomless sexually transmitted disease, she may inadvertently push the infection from the cervix up into the uterus.[25]

Further blurring the boundary between emergency contraception and therapeutic abortion is mifepristone, which used to be known as RU 486. It has just been licensed in this country, and has been received with suspicion by both the pro-life and pro-choice camps, the former because it is an abortifacient, and the latter because it is using women as guinea pigs for an under-researched drug. It has now been suggested that it is an effective form of emergency contraception although it is not being used in Britain in this way yet. We shall be discussing mifepristone later when we look at abortifacients.

Abortion For the Unwanted Pregnancy

Abortion is never recommended as a form of family planning, but rather as a last resort for some when all else fails. However, abortion figures in the West and, even more markedly, in some parts of the developing world where abortion is legal, would indicate that many people take more risks precisely because there *is* a fall-back method. We would venture to suggest that the abortion rate is high also because people have never been able to be as utilitarian *vis-à-vis* contraception as doctors and family planning agencies would like: we have explored this idea elsewhere. There has been an almost continuous increase in the abortion rate in this country since 1977: 'controversy' is not a large enough word to describe the public debate this has caused. Although it is legal with the permission of two doctors under certain circumstances up to twenty-four weeks, most abortions are performed in the first twelve weeks (and these are the easiest and safest). One reason for a late termination is the discovery by amniocentesis of a genetic defect: this is because the test cannot be done until sixteen weeks, and the results do not come in until three or four weeks later. We will be considering this in the next section.

The UK legal criteria for terminations are:

1. Continuing the pregnancy would involve risk to the life of the woman greater than if the pregnancy were terminated.

2. Termination is necessary to prevent grave permanent injury to the physical or mental health of the pregnant woman.
3. Pregnancy is not past week twenty-four and continuing would involve risk, greater than if the pregnancy was terminated, or injury to the physical or mental health of the woman or her existing child(ren).
4. There is a substantial risk that, if the child were born, it would be seriously handicapped, physically or mentally.

All women or couples need information and counselling before they proceed with an abortion. The session should be unhurried and ideally more than one session should be offered in order to allow space for reflection away from a medical environment. If accompanied, a woman should be offered an individual session in case she is being pressurised by her family or partner to have a termination. If she decides to proceed with the abortion, she also needs to be counselled about future family planning.

The type of abortion is determined by gestation. If a woman is less than twelve weeks pregnant, she is usually offered a surgical abortion. This is an operation that is usually done under general anaesthetic. During the operation, the cervix is dilated and the uterine contents evacuated by powerful suction. Although complications rarely occur, they include haemorrhage, perforation of the uterus and pelvic infection. Any of these may affect a woman's future fertility. Extremely rarely complications result in death.

Now we come once again to mifepristone. A doctor in this country may offer this new and controversial abortion pill treatment to a woman who is certain she is less than nine weeks pregnant. She swallows three tablets under medical supervision. She is then monitored for two hours. If all is well, she can go home for forty-eight hours, during which time she may start bleeding. When she returns to the hospital for her second appointment, a doctor or nurse will insert a prostaglandin pessary high into the vagina. Prostaglandin stimulates contractions of the uterus and 'ripens' the cervix. The abortion occurs 'like a heavy period' about four to eight hours later. The size of the fetus at this stage is smaller than a two pence coin and is therefore not easy to distinguish. The woman is usually able to go home the same day. She has a follow-up visit about twelve days later. Complications of this method are heavy bleeding in about ten per cent of patients.[26]

Once a woman has taken the initial tablets, she cannot go back on her decision. That is why all patients must receive counselling before they receive the tablets – although we wonder whether bona fide counselling can take place under these circumstances, especially if it is to be offered by busy GPs in the future. We are also concerned at reports that some women change their minds between the two stages of treatment. There is likely to be a great increase in the chance of birth defects should they decide to proceed with a pregnancy under these circumstances.

If a woman is more than twelve weeks pregnant, the risks related to a surgical abortion increase considerably. Abortions after twelve weeks are therefore induced medically and require the woman to be admitted to hospital. Prostaglandin is administered as a vaginal pessary every three hours (up to a maximum of five times) until the abortion occurs. A woman remains awake throughout the procedure, which is like a 'mini labour'. Obviously, every individual experience is different, but in general this method of abortion is more painful and stressful than the type that requires a general anaesthetic, especially if the woman sees the fetus. This method is sometimes more acceptable to women who want to keep their abortion secret, because it does not require an overnight stay. Following an abortion every woman should be offered a check-up visit, advice on future family planning and counselling.

Abortion For the Wanted Pregnancy

We have discussed abortion for the 'unwanted' pregnancy, but what about abortion for the 'wanted' pregnancy? Due to tremendous advances in both technology and chromosomal analysis, it is now possible to screen pregnant women for many different abnormalities. Pre-natal diagnosis is appropriate for only a small minority of women and the chances for most pregnant women of having an abnormal baby are very small.

To embark on pre-natal screening *presumes* that a woman would contemplate an abortion should an abnormality be likely.

However, the following groups are considered to be at increased risk. The list is not comprehensive, but it illustrates the complexities a 'high-risk' woman will have to grapple with as she sets out to make the 'best' decision.

1. Healthy women over thirty-five years old with no other risk factors have an increased risk of a baby with Down's syndrome. If a woman has had a previous Down's baby, her risk of another is 1 in 100 or greater depending on age. If she has a close relative with Down's it is more complicated and tests on the affected side of the family decide her risks. The following chart gives risks for the general population based solely on maternal age:

Woman's age in years	Means risk of live-born Down's baby
25	1 in 1200
30	1 in 900
35	1 in 400
37.5	1 in 200
40	1 in 100
43	1 in 50

2. A woman who has a personal or family history of a condition that has been linked to a single gene disorder such as haemophilia, cystic fibrosis, some types of muscular dystrophy, sickle cell anaemia etc.
3. A man or woman who has a close relative with severe mental retardation or serious congenital abnormality.
4. A man or woman who has a personal or family history of spina bifida or anencephaly.
5. A woman taking anti-convulsants (drugs used for epilepsy) or warfarin.
6. A woman who is suspected of having an infection that causes abnormalities in the baby. Rubella is a common example.

Fertility Control: the Choices on Offer

The following tests are offered to the pregnant women who fall into the above categories. It is very important to realise that if you would never consider having an abortion there is possibly no point in proceeding with any of these investigations.

One of the tests, the AFP, (done at about sixteen weeks gestation) is a routine blood test. Some women have to actively ask not to have it because they don't want to know. In fact many women do not know what the 'routine' pregnancy tests are. In the age when HIV screening is controversial some would be surprised to discover they were routinely being tested for syphilis.

1. Ultrasound is a method of scanning the fetus by means of high frequency sound waves. The technique is normally painless although it can be slightly uncomfortable because in the early stages of pregnancy the woman must have a full bladder. It involves lying on an examination couch and having a small hand-held device moved around the lower abdomen. Sound waves are relayed from this device to a computer and the image of the area being scanned is projected onto a screen. An early ultrasound scan is important to confirm a woman's dates and will diagnose a multiple pregnancy. If there is a serious abnormality it may be detected.

2. Chorionic villus sampling (CVS) is a test carried out after eight to ten weeks of pregnancy. It is a test for chromosomal abnormalities such as Down's syndrome. The chorion villus is the developing placenta which grows from the same cells as the baby and therefore has the same chromosomes (inheritance factors). The technique involves passing a needle through the mother's abdominal wall into the uterus (a local anaesthetic is usually used to numb the skin). An ultrasound scan is done at the same time to allow the doctor to guide the needle accurately. The doctor aspirates a tiny sample of chorionic villi. After the procedure, a woman is advised to lie down for one hour, and advised to take things easy for the rest of the day. The added risk of miscarriage is one to two per cent above the normal risk.

3. The AFP (Alpha-fetoprotein) test is a routine blood test done at sixteen weeks which tests for spina bifida and Down's syndrome. Its

accuracy depends on a woman being sure of her dates. Sometimes the test gives a false positive because a woman's dates are wrong. At other times no reason is discovered. It is not as sensitive as the Maternal screening test for Down's syndrome.

A low level of AFP is sometimes associated with Down's syndrome. A high level of AFP will give the risk of a baby with spina bifida (a condition of variable severity involving the spine not developing properly) and anencephaly (a condition when the main part of the brain does not develop). The test is designed to identify those women at increased risk of either abnormality so they can be offered further appropriate diagnostic tests. If these conditions are suspected, a woman is then offered counselling and a detailed ultrasound scan and amniocentesis. Out of ten women with a raised AFP level, only one woman will have a cause found. For the remaining nine, there will be no abnormality though these women are more likely to have a small-for-dates baby. To quote the Oxford Department of Medical Genetics 'It is easy to underestimate the anxiety that abnormal test results in pregnancy can generate, even after an ultrasound and amniocentesis have yielded normal results.'[27]

4. The Maternal serum screening test is also known as the Triple Test or 'Barts test'. It is a blood test which measures the levels of three substances in a pregnant woman's blood. It is a test that is free in some areas of Britain but in other areas women have to pay. The levels of these three substances are used in combination with a woman's age to estimate her risk of having a baby with Down's syndrome. The substances are alpha-fetoprotein (AFP), unconjugated oestriol (uE3) and human chorionic gonadotrophin (hCG). The test is done between fifteen and twenty-two weeks, usually at about sixteen weeks from the last period. If the results are 'screen negative' it will mean you are at low risk for Down's syndrome. On average only about one in 2000 'screen negatives' will have Down's syndrome.

5. The Triple-Plus test or 'Leeds Test' measures the same substances as the Triple Test mentioned above but in addition it measures neutrophil alkaline phosphatase (NAP). The levels of

Fertility Control: the Choices on Offer

these four substances are used in combination with a woman's age to estimate her risk of having a baby with Down's syndrome. This is more accurate than the Triple Test, on average only one in 5000 'screen negatives' will have Down's syndrome.

If any of the women test positive to the tests mentioned in 3, 4 or 5 then they will be offered some of the further investigations mentioned below. But remember that on average only one in fifty screen positives have Down's syndrome.

6. Amniocentesis is a procedure done at about sixteen weeks gestation that involves passing a needle through the mother's abdominal wall into the uterus (a local anaesthetic is usually used to numb the skin). An ultrasound scan is done at the same time to allow the doctor to guide the needle accurately. The doctor withdraws a small sample of the amniotic fluid surrounding the fetus. After an amniocentesis, a woman is advised to lie down for one hour, and advised to take things easy for the rest of the day. The added risk of miscarriage is 0.5 to 1 per cent above the normal risk. (Half that of the chorionic villus sampling.) She continues to be at a higher level of risk for a week, and so she may feel more at ease if she limits her activities for longer than just one day. Many hospitals recommend this, although there is no official confirmation that it makes any difference.

There are two tests done on the sample: the first is on the amniotic fluid itself and the second is on the cells which were floating in the amniotic fluid. The amniotic fluid can be tested for AFP or for some biochemical disorders, and these results can be available quite quickly. As there are only a few cells in the amniotic fluid they have to be cultured before they can be accurately assessed. They take three weeks to be cultured so a result is not available for three to four weeks following the procedures – and sometimes up to six weeks. Obviously, this wait is stressful for the mother who is now often just over twenty weeks pregnant and feeling movement but still uncertain about whether she is going to continue with the pregnancy. If she has not announced her pregnancy so as to protect herself from censure and her existing family from distress in the event of a termination, she will also have practical difficulties. It is just possible to conceal morning-sickness and the other symptoms of a first trimester pregnancy, but concealing a pregnancy at twenty weeks can mean having to wear tents and be bent over double.

7. An ultrasound scan for structural congenital abnormalities is carried out between eighteen and nineteen weeks. It often needs to be this late because the fetus has to be large enough to allow adequate examination for the more subtle abnormalities. More obvious abnormalities, such as severe spina bifida, will be visible before this time. Some minor abnormalities of the face such as a cleft lip will only be clearly visible around twenty to twenty-two weeks.

If a woman decides to proceed with a termination because of an abnormality, she will need counselling and emotional support. 'Several studies have shown that early termination of an unwanted pregnancy is rarely accompanied by severe or persistent psychiatric problems. The situation is very different for termination of pregnancy performed after diagnosis of severe fetal abnormality. In this case the termination ends a wanted pregnancy, and is psychologically painful and distressing for the parents. It is preceded by a period of intense anxiety accompanying the process of prenatal diagnosis.'[28]

Any woman who has experienced problems such as those above should be offered follow-up counselling and advice about future risks of abnormalities. Information about pre-conceptual care and vitamin supplements to reduce the risk of neural tube defects should also be offered.

In fact the umbrella of fertility control is already extending backwards to cover pre-conceptual preparation. In the next section we will offer a brief outline of how couples are encouraged to care for their fertility.

How To Care For Your Fertility

Is there anything a couple can do to optimise their chances of conceiving and minimise their chances of needing any medical intervention? And having conceived, what can they do to optimise their chances of bringing a perfect, healthy child into this world?

'By taking the trouble to find out about pre-conception care, you have shown yourself to be a responsible parent of the future,' states a leaflet on pre-conceptual care.[29] In this section we will briefly describe the pre-conceptual advice being offered to couples today.

Although there are many beliefs about health care before conception, there is still very little hard knowledge. We consider it is important to have a well-informed, common-sense, healthy attitude to preparing for a pregnancy without going overboard about health precautions.

It is thought that some problems may be caused by the parents' health prior to conception, due to damage to the oocyte or sperm as they develop. We know that babies may be damaged by heavy smoking or drinking, certain drugs, poor diets and certain infections such as rubella, toxoplasmosis or listeriosis.

This does not mean that everyone who smokes or drinks has an unhealthy baby or that by being fastidious about health a perfect baby is guaranteed. We have been dealing with statistics in many sections of this book and if you can tip the balance slightly towards producing a healthy child by being careful for the months prior to a conception it makes sense. To prevent this information creating unnecessary anxiety because it reaches many unplanned parents too late, we would encourage them to look at the overall statistics and see that their chances of having a healthy baby are *very* high.

In general couples are advised to allow three to six months to get themselves healthy. A reasonable amount of exercise will help keep your muscles in good tone. Any woman who is markedly under- or overweight has a reduced chance of conceiving and it is worthwhile aiming for the acceptable body weight for height. If a couple are under considerable stress it is important to explore ways of reducing it. Relaxation techniques can be helpful.

Aim to eat a healthy diet with sufficient protein and plenty of fresh fruit and vegetables; variety is the key to a healthy, balanced diet. The wider the range of foods you eat, the more likely you are to eat all the nutrients that you need. Avoid any health supplements containing vitamin A because high levels have been shown to cause abnormalities in babies. Liver contains high levels of vitamin A and liver and liver pâtés should therefore be avoided.

All women are now advised to take folic acid (400 mcg daily) while they are trying to conceive and during the first twelve weeks of pregnancy. If a woman has had a child in the past who was born with a condition associated with folic acid deficiency she should take 4 mg of folic acid daily. Women who are epileptic and on medication that reduces the amount of folic acid in the blood are advised to do the same throughout pregnancy.

Try to avoid smoking or drinking alcohol excessively. Excess alcohol consumption in early pregnancy can cause fetal alcohol syndrome characterised by mental and physical problems. A maternal alcohol level as low as ten units a week (a unit of alcohol is equivalent to a measure of a spirit, a glass of wine, or half a pint of beer/cider) has been shown to be associated with an increased risk of miscarriage, low birth weight, congenital abnormalities, fetal distress in labour and a lower childhood IQ. Women who smoke in pregnancy have an increased risk of miscarriage and premature labour. Smoking often damages the placenta resulting in a low birth weight baby. In men excessive smoking and alcohol intake have been shown to have a detrimental effect on the sperm. In recent years epidemiologists have associated men who smoke with childhood cancer and birth defects in their offspring.

Try to avoid all medicines including herbal medicine and seek medical advice if there is a drug you have to take. Women on the oral contraceptive pill are advised to discontinue it one month before conceiving and to use another method of family planning. Illegal drugs lack any quality control and may vary in purity and strength, this makes them especially hazardous. If you are addicted to any drug, seek professional advice.

There are so many different types of chemical that may affect the oocytes, sperm or fetus that it is impossible to list them all. If you live or work near to any hazardous or polluted area that may affect your health it may be important to seek advice. There is a growing body of research that suggests that some chemicals affect the sperm and cause future problems such as miscarriage, birth defects and diseases in children.

It is important to be free of any infection before planning a pregnancy. Sexually transmitted diseases can cause problems with both the fetus and the newborn baby and it is important to seek

Fertility Control: the Choices on Offer

advice if you think you are at risk and have appropriate tests. If you consider you are high-risk for having contracted the HIV virus, we advise you to seek counselling about pre-conceptual HIV testing. If the HIV test is positive, it is very important to discuss the implications for the mother and the baby.

All women should check that they are immune to rubella (German Measles). Many women are routinely screened when they attend for family planning. A history of having had rubella or having had the immunisation as a teenager is not sufficient, and a blood test is the only way of being certain. If you need to be immunised against rubella, it is important to wait at least three months before conceiving because the vaccine itself can cause problems. Other vaccines such as mumps, measles, polio and yellow fever should be avoided if possible.

While pregnant, what extra precautions should a woman consider taking? We are not trying to make you over-anxious about catching infections, but it is sensible to take simple precautions to avoid infections that are known to affect a fetus. At the time of fertilisation an ovum weighs about five millionths of a gram. By twelve weeks it has increased its weight more than two million times to about thirteen grams. It is during this stage of incredibly rapid growth that a baby seems to be most vulnerable to problems.

Listeriosis is an illness caused by a bacteria called Listeria monocytogenes. Listeriosis is a mild flu-like illness which can result in miscarriage, stillbirth, or severe illness in the newborn baby. Listeria may be found in high concentrations in certain soft cheeses such as camembert, brie and the blue-veined varieties. These types of cheese should be avoided during pregnancy. Some pâtés contain high levels of listeria and to be on the safe side it is wise to avoid pâté when pregnant. Ready-cooked meals kept cold but not frozen may contain a low amount of listeria. It is better to reheat these dishes very well and not to eat them cold. Avoid coming into contact with sheep that are lambing, because sheep are sometimes infected with listeria.

Toxoplasmosis is a mild flu-like illness caused by a parasite called Toxoplasma gondii. It is found in raw meat, unpasteurised goat's milk or unpasteurised goat's milk products; unwashed, uncooked fruit and vegetables, and cat faeces. Toxoplasmosis infection in the fetus can cause problems with the eyesight and hydrocephalus which might cause brain damage. Pregnant women should take extra precautions when handling raw meat, fruit and vegetables. They should avoid eating undercooked meat and unpasteurised goat's milk products. They should also avoid coming into contact with any areas which might be contaminated with cat faeces.

These are all ways to optimise your chances of conceiving a healthy child. But what about the occasions when the odds are not in your favour? This happens when a man or woman has a serious condition that requires a treatment such as chemotherapy or radiotherapy. These treatments are likely to affect the testes or the ovaries. Nowadays many people believe that men in such a situation should be offered the opportunity to freeze sufficient sperm for future use, and that women should be able to request that a wedge section be taken from the ovary and frozen, with the hope that it could be re-implanted after recovery.

So there you have the full range of fertility controls on offer. Before we conclude this chapter, we would like to address the processes involved in decision-making and suggest a way of viewing the difficult and complex decisions we have to make when controlling our fertility.

When we have to make an important decision, it is often very difficult, so much so that it is impossible to reach a decision with which we feel comfortable. We would all accept that with any decision there are gains and losses to be made, and that one has to be reconciled with the losses in order to move in the direction of the decision. But the pressures in our complex world often paralyse us and so prevent us from reaching any decisions at all. We act in ways we later see as 'impulsive' or 'irrational'.

We would like to suggest that this impulsive behaviour is more understandable and logical than has been given credit. Our whole lives consist of evaluating a series of risks and making decisions based on knowledge and previous experience. Crossing a road could take all day if we were unable to act in this way.

Fertility Control: the Choices on Offer

But some decisions are very complicated. If we look at the huge variety of influences that are playing their part and see all the pressures surrounding a decision, what we see is a series of rhythms and different tones, each of a certain strength and persuasiveness, and influencing us in many different ways depending on our own mood and place in time and space. It is all very well for people to say 'Take a step back, go for a walk alone, separate yourself from the closest influences,' but it is not always easy to make a decision in a vacuum. If the pressures of your everyday life are those you have to requite with your ultimate decision, then it may well be easier to make the decision surrounded by those influences.

There is no utopian solution, but we would like to suggest that it is possible to be systematic about assessing these pressures and influences. We would suggest that rather than take on the whole lot at a time, it would be easier to immerse yourself in a small section of the whole and listen as well as talk to others and try to identify why people care about the action you are considering and how you feel about it.

Some of these sections may not be easy to address because they relate to influential people from the past such as your family or teachers. Each may have had a strong influence on you and it may still be very important to you not to offend them or their beliefs. In childhood we learn a complex pattern of rules, pressures and taboos. Although we are often not fully aware of the process, it is important to recognise that we sometimes behave in a certain way because of powerful early experiences.

Obviously, the dynamics of any individual decision are unique, but we suggest that many of the patterns of influence in people's lives are similar, although the strength of those influences will vary. Imagine you are at the centre of these influences and that the decision you have to make is one concerned with your fertility control. We will suggest a series of questions you could ask yourself in order to be able to review each section of the complex influences in turn.

As well as doing this exercise for yourself, we suggest you go through the questions again. This time, consider how any of the following people view your problem, and how your decision may affect them: (1) your partner; (2) your friends and peers; (3) people from your place of work; (4) various members of your family; (5) other experts, e.g. your teachers, health professionals, solicitors.

Knowledge
Have you accurate information about the advantages and disadvantages of taking this action? Are you being offered inaccurate or biased information, and if so why?

Psychological
How do you feel about this decision and are you able to communicate your feelings to others? How are your feelings influenced by other people? Are you trying to please someone else? Will you be able to cope with the losses involved in making this decision? Have you given yourself enough time to make this decision? Are you feeling like acting impulsively to rid yourself of the uncertainty involved in making this decision? How do you think you will view this decision five years from now?

Socio-cultural
Are you aware of society having any strong views about your decision? Does it matter to you if you act in a controversial way? Have you been influenced by any media items or pressure groups? Would you care about acquaintances knowing about your decision?

Moral/Religious
Does your decision fit in with your own code of behaviour? Are your past or present religious beliefs influencing your decision? Do you feel anxious or guilty about your decision?

The Ideal Future Self
Will your decision affect your future career? Are there any financial anxieties? How far ahead in life had you planned your life? Was this realistic? How strongly are your future plans influenced by ideal people who seem to plan everything perfectly? Have you idealised these people?

Vulnerable moments when individuals may act more impulsively than usual

Are you having a relationship crisis? Are you concerned about your age in relation to your fertility? Are you using more alcohol or drugs than usual because of this decision? Are you having to cope with considerable stress? Are you on holiday?

Conclusion

We have done what we threatened to do earlier, namely to bring under one umbrella a number of categories that are usually kept separate, so as to suggest a wider definition of fertility control. Like it or not, the term has come to mean not just limiting the number of children you have and allowing only wanted pregnancies to continue, but also controlling wanted pregnancies for unwanted defects.

The way forward is clear; its implications frightening to most people. 1993 saw, for example, the opening of the London Gender Clinic. By putting sperm into albumen, its owners claim, they can separate male sperm from female sperm, because apparently the male sperm swim faster. The clinic claims that it will not treat childless couples. All couples chosen must agree to opt for a child of the opposite sex to the child or children they already have. They must also (although surely this cannot possibly be legally binding) agree to carry the resulting pregnancy to term. Although the service providers stress the importance of individual choice, they have been quoted as saying that parents 'should not play God' and 'should not attempt the perfect child'. Certainly, many critics of the service claim that their method is so unreliable that there is no question of this problem emerging.

But if gender-determination becomes a reliable service that is available to the general public, would there eventually be an imbalance of the sexes? Listen to Professor Winston, who questioned the setting up of the clinic when interviewed by the *Observer*. He has himself been a pioneer of technologies for testing and implanting embryos in women with family histories of inherited sex-linked disorders. 'We offer a sex selection service for women from families with sex-linked, inherited illnesses such as Duchenne muscular dystrophy,' he says. 'However, we have found that a proportion of people who come are seeking this service for very questionable reasons. There are very serious questions about their attitude to children who could end up by being damaged and endangered, particularly if they are born with the sex that was not desired by the parent.' A researcher quoted in the same article said that when he was working in a clinic in Australia, 'a couple with three girls came to us wanting a boy. We tried, but it turned out female. The couple simply terminated it.'[30] According to Jonathan Glover, 'the slippery slope arguments need not concern us in the UK because we can always draw a legal line.' But as he went on to point out, the time to start thinking about regulation is now. It will be harder and harder to know where the line ought to be drawn as genetic research progresses. What happens, for example, if they isolate the gene for autism? It is already being suggested that a time may come when parents and their unborn children will have to be tested and passed as healthy and normal before being eligible for medical insurance. How much control will we have over our fertility once this has come to pass?

These are the problems to think about in the future. But before leaving the subject of fertility control, it is important to remember that there is one rapidly growing twilight zone that needs addressing rather more urgently. Up until twenty-four weeks' gestation, all fertility decisions are based on the assumption that the baby in question is not yet viable. After twenty-four weeks, the baby is deemed viable and so becomes an individual in the eyes of the law. The concept of fertility control is no longer applicable; the task at hand is the protection of a new life. Just think what a strain this sudden change of gears puts on the parents. As they cross this dividing line, they must leave behind their perfect plans, their pre-imagined families, their imagined omnipotence. Now, suddenly, they must make do with second fiddle. It is the child who comes first now, the unique and imperfect baby to whom all attendants must adjust. Most of us would say that is as it should be. But consider the paradox that emerges with medicine's ability to save ever younger babies.

The Special Baby Unit at John Radcliffe Hospital in Oxford will

Fertility Control: the Choices on Offer

treat any woman whose baby is twenty-three weeks' gestation or over. It will even become involved if the pregnancy is twenty-two weeks, as there is sometimes a problem with dates. What this means is that there is now a two-week overlap, with babies of the same gestation being saved in one part of the hospital, and terminated in another part, and with some of the babies saved being less healthy than the ones being disposed of. Of course it is not as simple as that – most pregnancies being terminated at this stage will be as a result of an abnormality, and a woman whose labour has been postponed through the administration of steroids will generally give birth to a baby whose lungs are stronger than the lungs of a baby born at twenty-five weeks whose mother has not received this treatment. But the rule of thumb for neonatologists does remain the gestation estimate. If they go to a woman who is in labour or having a Caesarian section at twenty-two or twenty-three weeks, they will resuscitate fully if they detect any signs of life. Although they will remain in close contact with the parents, they will be representing the needs and rights of the newborn child first. Again, this is as it should be. What's more, most of us who have children today are comforted by the news that medicine is able to help ever younger babies survive. But think for a moment what the experience does to the parents.

Imagine, if you will, a thirty-seven-year-old woman who has planned her first child by the book. She has used contraception responsibly until such a time as finances allow for a family. She has conceived as a result of a joint decision with her partner. She has taken good care of herself throughout pregnancy, and taken all the recommended genetic tests. Her every action is based on the assumption that her fertility is something she can and must keep under her control. Because of bureaucratic delays during the Christmas rush, she doesn't get the results for her amniocentesis until she is twenty-two weeks.

The results reveal that the baby is normal. Finally she can relax and enjoy her pregnancy, she tells herself, but then, unhappily, at twenty-three weeks, she gives birth to a premature baby. Most of us will have had another four months in which to accustom ourselves to the discovery that the rules governing fertility control are the mirror image of the rules governing a viable baby. What kind of bends do you go through if you have to make this shift in less than a fortnight? To put it differently, if a person has been brought up and educated to think of fertility as something that must and can be controlled, and babies as entities whose fates are to be decided on while they are still in the hypothetical, how well equipped are they to deal with a real baby who is fighting for its life?

Should parents have the right to decide whether their premature baby should receive full care? This question is especially fraught for those who have been told their baby may be disabled. How far should medicine pursue the goal of saving all these young lives? Dr Jill Thistle points out that this 'raises an ethical question with far-reaching implications. The twenty-four-week limit for abortion recognises very small babies' likelihood of surviving, but women have the right to terminate for fetal abnormalities after this stage in the pregnancy. Many decide to exercise this right after careful consideration of the implications of having a handicapped child.[31]

There is another problem we must look at, too. The fertility control philosophy is based on the assumption that there is something to be controlled. It therefore does little to prepare people for the possibility of infertility. But where there is a need, there is a branch of experimental medicine. We'll be looking at the advances in fertility treatments in the next chapter.

CHAPTER SEVENTEEN

HOW SERIOUS IS THE THREAT OF INFERTILITY?

It is generally agreed that if you take one hundred sexually active women who are not using contraception, eighty of them will have become pregnant within the year. Despite disturbing but vague reports about the average sperm count for men having halved over the past half-century (which men were tested? where? and in comparison to what fifty-year-old study conducted by whom?), the human race is still doing too good a job of regenerating itself. The average duration of fertility in females is longer than ever. Girls in the West reach puberty at eleven or twelve – a good three years earlier than they did a century ago. It is not uncommon for women to start their families in their very late thirties and early forties. But that is not the same as saying that any woman who chooses to wait that late will get what she wants. In *Backlash*, Susan Faludi pointed out, rightly, that fertility is often more greatly affected by a woman's diet, standard of living, and general state of health than it is by her age. In the US, middle-class white women over thirty were, in fact, more fertile than urban black women in their twenties – this being largely due to a pelvic infection called Chlamydia that was rife in that age group in inner cities.[1] But statistical games like this are like adding apples and oranges. Middle-class women over thirty may be more fertile than younger, less affluent, urban women, but it is important to remember each individual thirty-something's own fertility is on the decline. Most women will be fertile enough to have their target number of children even if they start after thirty or thirty-five, but if this same group had started trying for children in their twenties, fewer would have run into problems.

In this country there has been a trend over the last ten or fifteen years to have babies at an older age. Many more babies are being born to mothers in the twenty-nine to thirty-nine year bracket. But there has recently been a very slight rise in the number of babies born to women at or after forty although the figure for both 1976 and 1986 in England and Wales is 4,800. Carefully controlled demographic studies of England between 1550 and 1849 by Professor Trussell of Princeton University and Dr Wilson of the London School of Economics have shown a similar drop in fertility after forty in the age before 'choice', and more recent studies of Hutterites (a very fertile Protestant in-bred sect in the US), the Swedes (moderately fertile) and the Chinese (the least fertile) show that in all three groups, fertility declines sharply after forty.[2]

Older mothers-to-be can expect a high standard of antenatal care in this country. If they agree to genetic screening, they can also afford to worry less about Down's syndrome, spina bifida, and other problems associated with high maternal age. But the older you are, the more likely you are to have fertility problems. Some of these problems will be due purely to ageing: defective eggs, less frequent ovulation, problems with cervical secretions, a greater likelihood of damage to the fallopian tubes, hormonal imbalances leading to over-short luteal phases or troubles with implantation or miscarriages. Sometimes infections, diseases, surgery, chemotherapy, or radiation treatment will be the cause of infertility, and sometimes it is a direct result of contraception. As we have already mentioned, women coming off the combined pill sometimes have trouble ovulating. Those using the IUCD run the risk of infections that can block the fallopian tubes, while the progestogen-only pill can temporarily affect the type of cervical secretions.

Some estimates put the number of couples having some kind of fertility problem as high as one in six.

What are the most likely problems if you have stopped using contraception while sexually active and fail to become pregnant? You may not be having sex often enough, or not at the right time of the cycle. You may have a mistaken idea of when your fertile phase is. Or you may not be having the right kind of sex – some women who come in for investigation turn out to be virgins, some couples will have been striking the right positions, but not moving afterwards, and therefore never reaching climax, while other couples – and yes, we are talking about people with impressive degrees and large mortgages – will have been confusing the anus for the vagina.

Or you may be having stress cycles. There is a great resistance to the idea of stress cycles amongst many fertility experts – we feel that part of the problem is due to the vagueness of the term. But there has been research indicating that stress cycles may be quite common amongst the overworked and the underweight. High stress levels can lead to a woman having anovulatory cycles – or, if she does conceive, her post-ovulatory luteal phase is not long enough for the corpus luteum to generate enough progesterone to give the uterine tissue the right environment for implantation. This will mean that she miscarries, usually without having had indication of a conception, at about the time of her expected period.

How to put an end to stress cycles? Put on some weight, lighten the work load, go away on holiday, and do what you have to do to relieve anxiety. A balanced diet is important, and so is staying away from alcohol and drugs. It's all very easy – if you are aware that stress can lead to infertility. Unfortunately, the converse is also true. A woman with unrealistic expectations about getting pregnant very quickly after coming off contraception will be shattered if a baby does not appear after two or three months – and so upset that she starts having stress cycles. These will add to her waiting time – and make her even more convinced that she has serious problems, when in all likelihood, she doesn't.

How to avoid *this* vicious cycle? It is difficult for couples to learn or appreciate the importance of relaxation and humour when it comes to fertility problems. British biochemist Paul Entwhistle claims to have been able to help stressed infertile couples with hypnotherapy.[3] In the US, acupuncture has been found to be helpful. Even experts averse to the idea of stress cycles admit that anxiety does not expedite fertility treatment. It is better to become acquainted very early in the game with the various causes of and treatments for infertility – always bearing in mind that none of these problems are likely:

1. There can be problems with the ovary. Ovulation may not be occurring at all or occurring very infrequently. There are many distinct causes. It may be due to a hormonal imbalance, or to being underweight, sometimes caused by stress. It may possibly be due to previous use of the combined pill. As we have already pointed out, this last situation is particularly common amongst women who started the pill very early while their cycles were still anovulatory. It is possible to kick-start the ovaries with a reasonable dose of Clomiphene. It is not necessary any more to go to a clinic for this treatment – GPs may administer it themselves, but they must do some of the fertility investigation first or else it may make subsequent investigations for sub-fertility difficult. The ovaries can be impaired because they are covered with cysts – this is called polycystic ovary disease. It is a condition that is variable in severity and, if severe, needs careful management.

2. There can be problems with the fallopian tubes. The most common single cause of infertility is blocked fallopian tubes. Any pelvic infection or surgery can cause adhesions – this means the tubes get stuck together. Scarring also occurs, affecting the lining of the tubes and the cilia. Blocked fallopian tubes can sometimes be opened – through laser treatment and/or by squirting liquid up the tubes under pressure – but even when they're clear, they don't necessarily function normally. Any inflammation or damage here can impede the egg's journey into the uterus, thereby resulting in ectopic pregnancy, which will often require the surgical removal of the tube. We cannot emphasise enough the importance of protecting yourself from sexually transmitted diseases. The most common organisms causing pelvic disease are the gonococcal and chlamydial infections. If you ever think you may have a sexually transmitted disease, it is vital that both you and your partner are treated as soon

as possible. To reinforce this message we will leave you with this sobering thought from a WHO publication:

> 'Some seventeen per cent of women who have pelvic
> infection for the first time and are treated for it, subsequently
> develop tubal obstruction and infertility. This figure rises to
> fifty per cent if the woman has had three or more episodes of
> infection. The risk of ectopic pregnancy . . . a pregnancy
> that develops in the fallopian tube and which can be fatal . . .
> increases seven to ten fold after an episode of pelvic
> infection. In England and Wales, for example an annual total
> of 83,000 cases of pelvic infection in women can be expected
> to result in about 8,600 cases of infertility due to tubal
> obstruction and 2,750 cases of ectopic pregnancy.'[4]

3. There can be problems with the uterus. Very large fibroids can interfere with implantation. Very rarely a woman will have an unusually shaped uterus which may lead to problems. And then there is Endometriosis, that has been more recently (and inaccurately) dubbed the 'career woman's disease'. Endometriosis is a condition in which the lining of the uterus presents in other parts of the body – exactly how, no one quite knows. Patches of these cells appear around the fallopian tubes, the vagina, and elsewhere. A laparoscopy (an examination when a tiny telescope is placed in the pelvis and the area is examined by a surgeon) will show these sometimes as chocolate-brown areas, which proliferate under the influence of oestrogen and progesterone, gradually decrease with the decrease in the levels of progesterone, and then shed into the abdominal cavity, causing irritations and matting. Fine fibrous bands form adhesions that cause organs such as the uterus and the bladder to get stuck together. The condition is very painful – particularly at the time of the period. Most sufferers have mild cases that are not thought to affect fertility, but endometriosis accounts for twenty per cent of all cases of infertility.[5] Treatment ranges from nothing other than analgesics, to hormone treatment, to surgery, to IVF. The hormone treatment of choice is Danazol, a by-product of testosterone, which induces a temporary menopause. If a woman with severe and fertility-threatening endometriosis wants

to try for a baby, the routine is for her to take Danazol for six months, and then come off it for a month or two in order to try to conceive. Many gynaecologists are now questioning this treatment. Although pregnancy can alleviate endometriosis, it can return afterwards.

4. There can be problems with the cervix. Extensive surgery can knock out the mucus glands, which results in an acidic vagina without protective cervical secretions. Cone biopsies – which have now been replaced, incidentally, by loop excision – can result in bad scarring. The cervix may be incompetent and cause recurrent miscarriage. This last condition requires a stitch to be inserted in the cervix early in the pregnancy to enable the woman to take a pregnancy to term.

5. Sometimes the problem is with the cervical secretions. Either there is not enough mucus or the cervical secretions contain antibodies that attack and immobilise sperm. The post-coital test involves examining a woman within twelve hours of having intercourse in order to take a sample of the cervical secretions and examine them under a microscope. It is essential to time this test accurately to coincide with the fertile mucus pattern.

6. Vaginismus is a spasm of the muscles of the vagina which occurs when a woman is trying to have intercourse. There are many causes of this condition. Sometimes it is related to previous abuse or trauma to the area. At other times it is due to anxiety about having intercourse. Sometimes this is the reason for infertility, although the couple may be too embarrassed to mention the problem. If no abnormality is discovered on examination, the couple is offered counselling.

7. There can be problems with the sperm. Low or zero sperm counts can result from mumps, radiotherapy, hernia, or undescended testicles. Normal sperm counts can be significantly reduced by excessive alcohol consumption, smoking, marijuana exposure, medication, chemicals used to seal the upholstery of car seats, insecticides, tight jeans, and many other modern evils. Quality of sperm is as important as quantity. If too many of a man's sperm are abnormal or immobile, his fertility will be reduced.

Research in this area is beginning to step up, but it has long been a neglected field. The only recourse of couples who cannot have children due to low or zero sperm count used to be Artificial Insemination. Nowadays, those with low sperm counts can also try IVF.

8. Male impotence can be the problem. Although things are beginning to change, impotence was often overlooked as a factor during fertility investigations – or else it came out disastrously late. One doctor told us about an experience he had had: an angry man dragged his sobbing wife into the clinic, shouting that she had failed to produce a baby after three years, and shaming her in front of the nurses. First the doctor took a history of the wife. Then he asked to check the husband, who agreed with great reluctance. It turned out that his penis and testicles were pre-pubescent size.

Impotence, the inability to have or maintain an erection, can be due to diabetes, excessive drinking or smoking, age, beta-blockers, or psychological reasons (guilt, nervousness about performance, fear, and lack of enthusiasm for the supposed object of desire are but a few of these). Many can solve the problem without formal treatment just by changing their habits or their attitudes, but treatments do exist for the seriously afflicted. There are also surgical implants available now that can help men have erections. Many men swear by them; other men's experiences have been bad enough to make the headlines. One man in Florida sued his surgeon recently because his implant caused him to have erections ninety per cent off target.

How soon should a couple with suspected fertility problems seek help? The average sexually active fertile couple has a twenty per cent chance of conceiving a child in any given month. Most of them will have conceived within six months. Most doctors recommend waiting for a year or eighteen months before seeking medical assistance – unless the woman is already over thirty-five, there is already an indication that ovulation is not occurring or there are signs of endometriosis. Usually it is the woman who takes the first step, although ideally the couple should seek help together, as the causes of infertility are shared a third of the time, and another third of the time solely traced to the man.

The first thing the doctor will do is to take a full medical history of both the man and the woman. This will usually include questions about sexual habits so that the doctor can make sure that the problem does not arise from infrequent intercourse. (Some couples have intercourse so infrequently that the woman's chance of conceiving is very small.) There will also be a full physical examination, again usually for both the man and the woman.

It is important to check that a couple is having intercourse at the correct time of the cycle. Many women have never been taught about the fertile time and are not aware of their cervical secretions. A couple is encouraged to have intercourse during the time when the crystal clear stretchy secretions (fertile mucus) are present. This information is especially helpful to those women with infrequent or irregular cycles, and is often the only information needed to achieve a pregnancy.

The woman may be asked to keep a basal body temperature chart (BBT) for at least three months. As we have explained already, such charts are *not* for timing intercourse so that it happens at the time of ovulation, but they are useful in determining (always *after* the fact) if ovulation has taken place.

If the woman has had irregular periods, or no periods at all (amenorrhoea), hormonal tests will measure the blood levels of FSH, LH, prolactin, testosterone, and oestradiol. There is also a progesterone test to check for ovulation. In a twenty-eight-day cycle it should be checked at day twenty-one, but if a woman has a twenty-one- or a thirty-six-day cycle the test should be adjusted. In these cases, or in women who have irregular cycles, a chart of the basal body temperature can be extremely successful in assessing when the test should be done. Thus it helps avoid unnecessary confusion.

The post-coital test establishes if the woman's cervical secretions and the man's sperm are compatible. A day or two before ovulation, and about twelve hours after intercourse, mucus is taken from the cervical canal, placed on a slide with a grid and the sperm therein counted and their movement patterns noted. The number of sperm present in each microscopic area is counted and their movement through the mucus recorded. In a good test at least five sperm are seen in each area swimming actively in a straight line through the mucus. The most common reason for a poor post-coital test is wrong timing. If a woman understands the fertile pattern of cervical secretions, she will optimise her chances of having a satisfactory test.

An ultrasound scan will provide more accurate information about the size and position of the uterus and ovaries. In the uterus, it can diagnose fibroids and show the thickness of the endometrium (the lining of the uterus) as well as helping to detect hydrosalpinxes, which are collections of fluid inside the fallopian tubes indicating a blockage. It will also help determine the existence of any problems with the ovaries. The scan may be used to monitor the growth and maturation of the ovarian follicles and to observe ovulation.

A laparoscopy helps to determine the outside condition of the fallopian tubes and the uterus, and also to establish the existence and the extent of endometriosis. Usually under a general anaesthetic, a tiny incision is made below the navel, and a laparoscope is connected to a powerful light source that allows the doctors to look inside at pelvic organs. The procedure usually lasts between fifteen and thirty minutes.

A hysterosalpingogram is another method that detects blockage of the fallopian tubes. Dye is injected from the uterus, and then an x-ray is taken. If there is a blockage, the dye will not be able to flow through the fallopian tubes. The x-ray also yields useful information about the condition of the uterine cavity.

Some women have found this investigation both painful and distressing. If the hysterosalpingogram suggests an abnormality in the uterus, hysteroscopy is performed. This involves passing an endoscope, a tiny viewing device, into the uterine cavity to assess the problem.

Dilatation and curettage, more commonly referred to as a D and C, was often carried out routinely for investigating infertility. It involves a general anaesthetic. The cervix is dilated and the uterine lining is scraped and the scrapings are sent for analysis. Although it does detect some hormonal problems and endometritis (inflammation of the lining of uterus), its practical value is now open to question as a routine investigation.

Investigation of male infertility will usually begin with a doctor taking a full medical history of the man. This will include a full physical examination. Following this he will be asked to provide at least two sperm samples. He will usually be asked to abstain from sex for three days, and then to masturbate into a container. He should try to get this sample into the lab as soon as possible, preferably within the hour. The sample will then be assessed for the volume of the ejaculation, the acidity of the semen, the sperm density, the percentage of motile sperm, the number of white blood cells, and sometimes the presence or absence of sperm antibodies. Researchers are becoming increasingly aware that it is not the quantity of sperm that matters, but the quality. It is hoped that there will soon be a computerised way of assessing sperm and tracking healthy sperm movement patterns, as well as new staining techniques, which may give a more accurate assessment of the sperm.

Sometimes men with a consistently low sperm count (oligospermia) or an absence of sperm (azoospermia) have a blockage. In order to determine whether an operation will be helpful there is a set procedure. First a testicular biopsy (taking a tiny sample of the testes with a needle) is carried out, and if this indicates that normal sperm production is occurring then the man may be asked to undergo surgical exploration of the testicles, the epididymis and the vas deferens. The tubes being opened are very small and new microsurgical techniques are offering improved results in restoration of fertility.

Occasionally, a consistently low sperm count or absence of sperm will be due to hormone deficiency. To find out if this is so, blood levels of testosterone, FSH and prolactin are carried out. If a hormonal abnormality emerges it is sometimes treatable, although the overall success rate of improving fertility is poor.

There is no established order in which these tests are performed, and not all tests are necessary for all couples. The key (and a key that is easy to lose in the wilderness of technical jargon) is common sense: a good doctor or a good clinic will make sure all the reproductive organs and identifiable processes have been assessed – especially if there is an idea to proceed to IVF, GIFT, or one of the other methods of assisted conception. About fifteen per cent of all couples seeking treatment will have what is called 'unexplained fertility'. Professor Winston feels this figure would be much lower if fertility investigations were more thorough and more rigorous standards were upheld.

If the problem turns out to be a low sperm count, or no sperm count at all, and it can be traced back to impaired sperm production, there is, at present, very little that doctors are able to do. In the event of a proven hormone deficiency, hormone treatment will sometimes work. If the sperm count is low but not too low, IVF is becoming an increasingly popular option. If the sperm count is low to zero because of a blockage, on the other hand, it may be relieved surgically.

Hormonal patterns account for twenty to twenty-eight per cent of all infertility cases. If a woman turns out not to be ovulating due to hormonal imbalances, there are various forms of treatment open to her. As we have already mentioned, Clomiphene can help many women to start or resume ovulation. If a woman has low-weight-related amenorrhoea, she will be asked to gain weight. If polycystic ovaries have been found, she will be asked to lose weight in addition to being given hormone treatment. Other disorders, such as hypergonadotrophic hypogonadism, hypopituitarism, and hyperprolactinaemia, respond to hormone treatment. Sometimes surgery will be recommended for hyperprolactaemia if drug treatment fails. Congenital abnormalities may sometimes be corrected with surgery.

If a woman has blocked fallopian tubes (this accounts for twenty-two per cent of all cases), it may be possible to unblock them using surgery. In addition she can undergo a procedure called adhesiolysis salpingolysis, which attempts to divide adhesions, i.e. separate organs that have become stuck to one another. Or else (if both ends of her tubes are open) she can have the healthy ends of her tubes joined together with the help of microsurgery. This last procedure has become increasingly popular and successful in recent years.

If no simpler solution exists, a couple can consider in-vitro fertilisation (IVF). Here we enter a new arena, where costs are high, results still very much on the low side, procedures often at the experimental stage, and standards, both for treatment and for eligibility, still blurry and controversial. There are at present forty-two clinics offering IVF in the UK: two are fully funded by the NHS, while seventeen are linked to the NHS – this means that NHS patients are subsidised by private patients. The great majority of patients receive treatment at the twenty-three private clinics. Costs range from about £1,000 to £2,000 per course of treatment. About 7,500 women sought IVF treatment in the UK in 1988. Success rates are difficult to assess. Although one study has indicated that twenty per cent of couples can benefit from IVF treatment, younger people attending the better-run clinics have a far better chance of success than do older people or people attending the less well-run clinics. When you read about success rates, make sure you know what age groups the patients fall into, whether they are talking about the conception rate or (considerably lower) the live birth or 'take-home baby' rate, and whether they disclose how many of those take-home babies came from multiple births. (The chances of a multiple pregnancy with IVF are twenty-four per cent, as opposed to one per cent for the general population; the chances of an ectopic pregnancy are five per cent, as opposed to the normal one per cent.) Another term to watch out for is the cumulative rate, which, again, will be much higher than the rate per cycle of treatment. To illustrate this with some figures, the conception rate for under thirty-fours with one cycle of treatment is twenty per cent. With three cycles it is forty-one per cent, and with five cycles it is fifty-five per cent. The cumulative live birth rates for the same age group are lower: thirteen per cent for one cycle, thirty-three per cent for three cycles, and forty-five per cent for five cycles. These figures drop roughly by a third for the thirty-five- to thirty-nine-year-old group, and by yet another third for the forty- to forty-five-year-old group. Although they will, as a rule, be better the better the clinic, all clinics show a drop in success with an increase in the patient's age.[6]

It is also important to bear in mind that most clinics have other entrance requirements. These are not standardised, but may include a doctor's assessment of the patient's motivation and psychological health. Single or unmarried women cannot expect to be welcomed, and may find themselves obliged to seek help from the private sector.

To return to the treatment itself: IVF involves the removal of one or more eggs from the ovary, the collection and purification of sperm, the mixing of sperm and egg in a laboratory, and then, if fertilisation occurs, the insertion of the developing embryo into the uterus, usually two or three days later, at the four to eight cell stage. It is meant to be offered as a last resort, when tubal surgery has proved unsuccessful, or has less of a chance of success than IVF. It has been proven useful when the man's sperm count is low, but not too low, when a woman who is still ovulating has been suffering from endometriosis, when there is evidence of cervical hostility to the man's sperm, when there are two or more serious problems in the same couple, when the woman is the beneficiary of egg donation following premature menopause, and also in cases of unexplained infertility – although this should only happen if the couple has already been thoroughly investigated.

IVF is no help if the woman is not ovulating despite stimulating the ovaries with the drugs previously described – unless she has opted for egg donation. It is also useless after she has had a hysterectomy, if she has severe uterine abnormalities, uterine tuberculosis, scarred or cystic ovaries, or severe bowel adhesions, and is inadvisable if she is much over forty-two years of age.

Here are the stages of treatment: (1) a suitability assessment, which involves physical or sometimes other types of tests; (2) the stimulation of the ovaries with drugs to get several follicles to develop; (3) the monitoring of the follicles' growth; (4) the collection of the eggs two to three hours before ovulation, either by laparoscopy or, more usually, with the help of an ultra-sound scan; (5) sperm collection, washing, and counting; (6) the establishment of an egg culture – after the eggs have been identified under a microscope, they are placed in a culture medium in an incubator, and then the sperm is mixed into the fluid containing the egg; (7) the establishment of embryo cultures – after eighteen hours they are checked to see if fertilisation has occurred, and at forty-eight hours, when they should be at the two to four cell stage, they are checked again for morphology; (8) the embryos are transferred to the woman – up to three fertilised eggs are loaded into fine plastic tubing with a tiny drop of culture fluid, and, after a vaginal examination, the tubing is inserted into the cervix and the fluid containing the embryos squirted gently into the uterus. Some clinics follow this up with an injection of progesterone to help with implantation.

Very occasionally the drugs that are given to stimulate the ovaries result in 'hyper-stimulation syndrome'. If it is severe, it may require hospitalisation.

Some clinics will also have frozen any embryos they have not used for future purposes. The general (and somewhat controversial) practice these days is to transfer more than one fertilised egg at a time to the woman because this increases the chances of a conception occurring, but current licensing regulation in this country puts the maximum at three.

Seven, twelve, and sometimes fourteen days after the embryo transfer, blood is taken and then tested on day fourteen for evidence of pregnancy. If no pregnancy has occurred, you can choose to have another course of treatment. Some clinics recommend trying at least three times, with two to three months' rest in between cycles. Many clinics set no limit to the number of times you can try, and others do set a limit – again, there are no set rules. Some couples have had more than ten treatments.

As some clinics get much better results than others, it is useful to know what makes a clinic less or more effective. According to Professor Winston, a good clinic does not accept self-referral, does communicate with the referring GP, does request and review all previous records, offers no treatment before a full investigation, performs the tests as rapidly as possible, ensures a full range of tests at all times, offers comprehensive treatment and continuity of care as well as free counselling independent of hospital treatment, shows a willingness to review results without charge, and offers pregnancy testing on site plus any necessary follow-up. A good clinic will also accept failure. It can say: 'It's not worth your while.'

A bad clinic (again according to Professor Winston) has an all non-NHS staff, offers immediate treatment without investigation, is equipped to provide or promotes one type of treatment rather than a comprehensive range, misquotes its results, dumps patients in an emergency, keeps on offering treatment regardless, and does not accept failure.[7]

GIFT, or gamete intra-fallopian transfer, is an alternative form of assisted conception suitable for women with patent (unblocked) fallopian tubes. The first steps are the same as for IVF. Instead of combining the egg and the sperm in a laboratory, they are drawn separately into a fine catheter and transferred into the fallopian tube. Again, the number of eggs transferred is usually no more than three, with the excess eggs generally being fertilised and then frozen. The egg and sperm transfer procedure takes between thirty minutes and an hour. The main drawback of the method is that fertilisation cannot be confirmed. Although the overall pregnancy rate of GIFT has been quoted as 21 per cent, the likelihood of that pregnancy being part of a multiple birth is 31 per cent. If a woman with triplets is counted as having three pregnancies, then you could see that the figures for success would look very different if they counted pregnant women rather than pregnancies.

Other new forms of assisted conception, all variations on IVF and GIFT, and most still too new to have yielded reliable success rates, are POST, DIPI, ZIFT, PROST, TET, TEST, and DOT. Hardly a month passes without a new acronym for assisted conception appearing. Micro manipulation is another experimental method that is being used in cases of severe male infertility where IVF has failed. A micro manipulator is a device which greatly magnifies the egg, allowing a specialist to strip the egg of its outer cells, position it on a pipette and then either make a small opening for the sperm to pass through or inject the sperm directly into the egg. At present, it has a low success rate, but there are high hopes for the future.

Artificial insemination with the husband's semen (AIH) is suitable for couples who have severe trouble with intercourse, or where the man wants to bank his sperm prior to chemotherapy. This involves introducing the semen directly into the vagina and the cervix. If it is introduced into the uterus, it is called IUI. This is useful if there are cervical problems. It is not useful where the man has a low sperm count unless it is used in conjunction with super-ovulation (i.e. hormone treatment to stimulate ovulation).

Artificial insemination by donor (AID), also known as 'Donor insemination' (DI) is appropriate where the man has no sperm or where there are genetic reasons for not using his sperm. It is often the only option open to unmarried women who want to have children – although again, many clinics refuse to treat women who are not in 'stable, happy marriages or relationships'. This is often a euphemistic way of saying that they will not accept lesbians.

The method is fairly straightforward. A good centre will take a full medical history as well as doing a full physical examination. It will monitor ovulation, with a view to performing the procedure just before ovulation occurs. After examining the cervix with a speculum, a semen sample is injected into the cervix. The procedure is meant to be painless.

Sperm banks can keep sperm for years at minus 196 degrees centigrade. Information about donors is confidential. Donors must undergo rigorous medical tests. Since the advent of AIDS, fresh semen is no longer used because, to make sure the sperm is free of the virus, the donor has to have two AIDS tests, one before the donation, and another six months later. No sperm is used until the all-clear after the second test.

Children born as a result of artificial insemination by donor to a married woman in the past were considered legitimate, although the legal concept of legitimacy no longer exists after the Children's Act of 1989.

Most women will not have to avail themselves of the new assisted fertility treatments – or will decide that such procedures are too stressful, costly, and unreliable to be worth trying. Even so, it's good to have some idea somewhere in the back of your head about how much time you would need if you or your partner really did have problems serious enough to warrant IVF treatment. We asked one specialist when a woman who definitely wanted children would be wise to test her fertility in order to take full advantage of current treatments if the need arose. He said that if she's hoping to have two, she should start trying at thirty-one or thirty-two. Most doctors recommend trying for a year or even longer before beginning investigations. This will bring her up to the age of thirty-three. Although some specialists are now working out ways to speed up these procedures, the average time for investigations is a year. This will mean she is thirty-four years old when she puts herself forward for IVF treatment. The average waiting list is about a year, which will make her thirty-five when she has her first course of treatment. Although the statistics are not in her favour (as we have shown, success rates are highest for the under thirty-four age bracket), she still has a far better chance of the treatment working at thirty-five than she would five years later, so let us assume that she gets pregnant on the third try. (We are also assuming, of course, that she can afford the treatment.) By the time she conceives, she is thirty-six. She is thirty-seven when she gives birth. She will have to think carefully about whether or not to breast-feed and, if she does so, about how long she should continue. For most women, lactational amenorrhoea is a plus, but for this woman, it could be a waste of valuable time. If she wants that second child, she should start up a new course of IVF treatment fairly soon, because the success rate is not good for the over forties.

The Debate about Pregnancy in Middle Life

In 1990 there were only fifty-eight women who gave birth after the age of fifty.[8] There are a variety of reasons why fertility declines so much earlier than the menopause, which occurs on average at around fifty to fifty-two years.

Middle-aged couples tend to make love much less frequently, which would naturally result in falling fecundity.[9]

Irregular cycles occur increasingly frequently as women become older.

There is a link between fertility and the age of the male partner.

- Most women are married to men older than themselves and, although male fertility does not decline so sharply, men are prone to produce an increased number of defective sperm after the age of forty-five.
- Older women produce more defective oocytes which result in more miscarriages.
- Older women have more fibrous tissue in their uterine muscle and are more prone to fibroids, which are sometimes associated with infertility.
- The endometrium (the lining of the uterus) may be abnormally thick, which may interfere with implantation.

Despite all these problems, many women, as we have seen, are postponing child-bearing, and therefore an older group of women, if unsuccessful, are actively seeking help from infertility clinics. Unfortunately, for the reasons stated above, the chances of a woman over the age of forty conceiving with the help of IVF and having a baby to take home are substantially less than in women less than thirty-five years old. The main reason is thought to be due to the older oocyte.

Recently there has been considerable interest in the use of oocyte donation from younger women with healthy oocytes to older women past their menopause. A recent report by Sauer[10] has shown that it is possible for women over the age of fifty to give birth following this procedure. Many people are now questioning whether this is a sensible use of medical technology.

There is also a heated debate about the suggested use of eggs from aborted foetuses. There are two issues here. One concerns elderly parents. The other concerns the wisdom of creating children for 'parents' who never lived. The possible misuses of this future technology are obvious and terrifying and make the problems of an older mother seem benign. One notices that the debate here seems to be focused on the selfishness of the woman. It seems to be an accepted part of our culture that some men choose to father children late in life.

Professor Winston comments:

> 'Research shows that children fare the best with a caring parental relationship and this may not be forthcoming as parents get older and less able to supervise a vigorous,

growing youngster. Becoming a parent is more emotionally stressful and physically demanding than many infertile couples appreciate and, although pregnancy is commenced with the best intentions, the arduous nature of having a baby when one is in middle-age may not be fully realised by couples considering oocyte donation. Also the risks of pregnancy are very considerable in women over the age of fifty years, and the desperation of a menopausal patient to have children should not override the real need for the most careful counselling in such circumstances.

Above all, medical practitioners should not forget that the menopause is a natural biological event. Perhaps we devalue the considerable advantages of ageing and maturity by trying too hard to circumvent the end of reproductive life in this way. When complex and expensive technology is used for social rather than pathological reasons, we cross what may be a dangerous boundary and promote risks which are genuinely unjustified.'[11]

In response to the controversy surrounding a pregnant sixty-two-year-old Italian, some people are calling for the Human Fertilisation and Embryology Authority (HFEA) to set an age limit for recipients of donated oocytes. Professor Ian Craft, director of the London Fertility and Gynaecology Centre, has urged moderation: 'Pregnancy occurs naturally, albeit rarely, up to the age of fifty-five. I would support egg donation until this age.'

The oldest mother at Professor Craft's centre was forty-nine years old. She gave birth to twins. All requests for assisted conception at the centre are considered by an ethics committee of fourteen people including theologians and lawyers.

Professor Craft considers that ovum donation is technically easy in post-menopausal women, as the uterus is in a stable state and can be stimulated by the correct dose of oestrogen and progesterone.[12]

Each couple have their own personal story and reasons for pursuing the often frustrating route of late parenthood. The best guideline a couple can use is to consider the consequences before, and not after, they take a chance.

The answer to the question we posed at the beginning of this chapter, then, is that there's no real need for most of us to worry about infertility, but that if we know about the treatments on offer, we will be better equipped to make more realistic plans and put any problem we might encounter into perspective.

CHAPTER EIGHTEEN

AND FINALLY –
THERE'S NO SUCH THING
AS A MISTAKE

This is not to say it's all plain sailing, either. To illustrate our point, let us return to Jack and Jill, whom we left, you will remember, basking in the glow of a rational decision. Let's imagine that three months have passed without the pre-planned blessed event occurring. They – although perhaps we shouldn't say that, because, as you will remember, Jack is not quite as keen on this idea as Jill is . . . so let's just talk about Jill for the time being. Jill has gone from smugness to distressed surprise to uncertainty to incipient panic. What's wrong with her? she wonders. She's been doing everything right, so where's her mistake?

Because she's too ashamed to talk to a friend, she finds herself in a bookstore while taking an extended lunch hour from that job that you will remember she was looking forward to leaving in the event of a pregnancy. There, in the mother and baby and women's issues corner, she finds this book. She calls in sick, takes it home, reads the first twelve chapters, and is so depressed by their contents that she finds herself unable to turn another page. Jack returns home from work to find her lying like a lump of unsorted laundry on the bed. He asks her what's wrong. She hands him the book. It looks like just the type of 'women's' book that sends him straight to sleep. But there are gale force winds that night, and they contrive to interfere with television reception. Bored and restless and hoping that things will change so that he can watch 'Match of the Day', he finds himself skimming the book, and then slowing down to read the sections he is worried might pertain to himself with growing horror. Before long he is lying inert and despairing in bed alongside, his inert and despairing and lightly moaning wife. Although this happens to be one of the days designated for procreative intercourse, neither of them can find the will to lift a finger.

All the things they didn't know! they say to themselves, and eventually, as the days roll on, to each other. How fragile and fallible our reproductive systems! How fallible the so-called miracle treatments! How makeshift our best-laid plans! How distressing the suggestion that our desire for children is not just irrational, but does not always translate into a love of offspring! And how painfully true that other suggestion that no baby is ever fully wanted, that a joint decision can be a cover-up, concealing the truth that one party wants it a good deal more than the reluctant other.

But one good thing has come out of all this dreariness. It has drawn Jack and Jill closer to each other, made it possible for them to talk to each other about their feelings. Which is good, Jill says, because they were drifting apart, weren't they? Encouraged by the new atmosphere of openness, and made reckless by Jill's attention, Jack now makes the dreadful mistake of mentioning in passing his ill-advised and ultimately empty office affair. The moment the words come out of his mouth, he wants to kick himself. What he had been trying to do was explain why he felt he had no right to object to Jill's proposal to start their family – because he felt so guilty about his philandering. But couldn't he have made up a less hurtful imaginary example to put across the same idea?

Jill takes the news badly. They have an ugly argument. She packs his bags for him. He isn't even as far as the car door before she is outside in her dressing gown, begging for him to come back. That night they have their best sex in years. Jill is absolutely sure that this time she has conceived. She can feel it in her bones, she says, but as it turns out, she is wrong. This time, when her period arrives, they both cry, because Jack's feelings have changed now. During the half-minute or so that he spent standing outside his house with his suitcase that night, thinking that their marriage was over, he, too, had realised that he wanted a child – a son! – more than anything, anything! in the whole wide world.

There's No Such Thing as a Mistake

And now it has been four months of failed attempts. 'Well,' he tells Jill tearfully, 'where there's a will there's a way.' They know from their new bible that it's far too early for them to be worrying, and that the stress of failure could be adding to their problems. 'Let's give ourselves six more months,' Jack suggests. 'Let's not even hope for anything to happen before then. In the meantime, however, I think we would be well-advised to get some professional advice about those temperature charts, because it could well be that your cycle is a departure from the norm.' 'Oh Jack!' gushes Jill, 'I can never get over how practical you manage to be in a crisis!' She generously neglects to mention that she herself has begun to wonder if the real problem doesn't lie in his sperm count.

And so one month turns into another. Before long, they are taking their long-planned trip to Australia. A holiday will do the trick, they think. By the time they discover that it hasn't, they have both turned into fertility bores. By June – Baby's original projected due date – it has become so bad that even their dearest friends dread having to invite them over for supper. They can't seem to talk about anything else. They have this embarrassing habit of asking other couples if their children are planned, or, if they don't have any yet, when they plan to have them, and whatever these other people say, Jack and Jill will exchange sad, smug smiles, as if to say, 'When will these people see the light? When will they realise that they are their own worst enemies?' They'll launch into boring and usually inappropriate lectures about 'the language of choice' or the 'politics of fertility' or 'the spectre of eugenics in the family planning movement' – things which no one else at the table would ever want to talk about. And, if the host at one of these unfortunate gatherings tries tactfully to change the subject, they'll go on the offensive. 'You think you have all the answers,' Jill will say to the woman sitting opposite. 'Well, then, tell me. How long is the normal woman fertile during any one cycle?' Having procured the desired wrong answer, Jack will say, 'If you don't even know that, how can you pretend to make an informed decision?' 'And how can *you* presume to say,' Jill will exclaim, turning towards the man to her right, 'that abortion should be made harder to get rather than easier. Are you meaning to tell me that you would feel that way if it were your daughter who was pregnant?' 'Yes,' Jack will add, 'and how about if you found out your wife were pregnant by your next-door neighbour?'

During the ensuing argument, Jack's closest friend is heard to say to Jack, 'You may be right about everything, you may well be right. But I swear, if you mention that damned book to me one more time, I'm issuing a *fatwa*.' But it doesn't come to that, because as it turns out (ironic, isn't it?), Jill is already pregnant at the time of the argument. As the pregnancy progresses, they develop new obsessions, and soon become embarrassed about their old ones, and they begin to wonder if it helped them at all to read that book and subject themselves to that crash course in fertility. Now that they have the outcome they wanted, their sense of perspective has returned. And they say to each other, after all, it only took us nine months. . . .

To which we say, yes, a little extra learning is a dangerous thing, especially if you are already in a crisis. We would also like to apologise to Jack and Jill's friends for the evenings our book may have ruined. There is only one thing worse than an instant expert, and that is two of them at the same table. There are many good reasons for keeping fertility off the list of acceptable subjects for polite conversation. But there are, we believe, even more reasons for people to arm themselves with a better general understanding of fertility before they even begin to think about what they themselves want to do. We realise we have only exacerbated Jack and Jill's problems in the short run, but we hope that the questions our book has raised will make them think and ask questions about their own attitudes to fertility, and so help them approach future crises more temperately.

At which point we would like to spell out our understanding of fertility awareness. It is not knowing how 'a' body works but how *your* body works, not going solely by what your doctor means by fertility, but also finding out what other things your fertility means to *you*. It is seeing risks you take and the choices you make not just in terms of politics and ethics and public health statistics but in terms of your own life story. It is never presuming that you know enough about someone else's life story to step in and make 'the best decision' for them. And, probably most important, it is ceasing to allow the fertility professionals more and more room for expansion, intrusion and regulation by ceasing to mystify their power. Even the most ardent critics of reproductive technology have a way of exaggerating their power by casting them as the big bad patriarchs. The fertility professionals will cease to have the upper hand the day we make their business our business, the day we stop going to them for the answers to our questions and see first how well we can answer them ourselves.

By which we are not saying that medicine is evil – after all, one of us is a doctor – but that it is, like all institutions, best kept within limits, and that we, the so-called consumers, are perfectly able to understand enough of what doctors are doing to be able to have an opinion. Medical knowledge is not as abstruse as we tend to think. When we say we can build up our powerbase and safeguard our rights by asking questions, though, we don't just mean asking questions about public policy. We mean asking questions about our own lives. Questions like: 'Why do I find this decision so frightening?' or, 'What is the difference between my understanding of this problem as a woman, and his understanding as a man?' or, 'How much responsibility *should* a man take? How much say do I want to let him have?' or, 'How much of that discussion I just had with my partner was about a baby, and how much of it was about the problems the two of us happen to be having at this particular moment?' or, 'Why did I take that stupid risk? And ought I to have said "we"?'

Not that we would wish a frivolously calculated risk, or its consequences, on anyone. But it's important to remember that it happens to the best of us. You don't believe us? We'll leave you with a true story that will have Jack and Jill and all other readers who have found themselves in a similar predicament laughing all the way to the delivery room.

We are not going to say where the confession comes from. Suffice it to say that the culprit could be one of the authors of this book, and that it goes without saying we are not talking about the one who's a doctor.

Imagine now an educated woman with all the latest information on fertility at her fingertips, and not only that. Also at her fingertips is the typescript of a book on fertility to which she is adding the finishing touches. She has three children, two step-children, big bills, and no steady income, but sometimes she fantasises about having another child, a somewhat urgent fantasy because she is forty. She suspects her partner also wants a child, but of course he would never come out and say that, would he? Although she has interviewed too many men on fertility to shrug her shoulders blithely, in the manner of so many women she interviewed, and say, 'Men are just like that' . . . she happens to know that *this* man is.

She knows from her book that most people are mysteriously superstitious about fertility, and that is one of the reasons why they don't bother to get the facts. She herself does have the facts, but she is still superstitious. She knows that if she waits a year, as her partner has now suggested, and plans a child, she might not get what she wants. So she becomes casual about contraception. Better that a baby comes early, she says to herself, than not at all. It is only after she finds out she is pregnant that it occurs to her that it would also have been better if she had been clear to her partner about her intentions.

But this is jumping ahead of the story, because it takes her a very long time to even admit to herself that she is pregnant. This failure to read the symptoms is one more thing to be embarrassed about when she finally faces the fact that she is three months pregnant. One of the things that has become clear to her through talking to women who have had abortions is that it is a very bad idea to have an abortion because you think other people will want you to have one, even if you know that if it were left to you, you wouldn't. Nevertheless, the first thing she says to her partner when she breaks the news to him is that she will have an abortion if that's what he wants, even though she herself doesn't.

He accuses her of putting him in an invidious position. Discussions get off to a very bad start. Our culprit continues to make every mistake in the book – by which, you will remember, we possibly mean this book. As she battles with morning-sickness to retouch

There's No Such Thing as a Mistake

those last finishing touches, time and time again, she breaks down, sobbing, 'Why am I incapable of following my own advice?' It is not until long after the optimum time for an abortion has passed, that she tragically decides to have the baby anyway, despite her own acknowledged errors of judgement. Her reason? 'I made a mistake, and now I'll have to pay for it. I won't make the baby pay for it, because it's not the baby's fault.' Even as she strikes this pose, she realises, guiltily, that this is a wonderful way of looking noble when actually, when it comes down to it, and as her partner has suggested, what's really happened is that she's getting her own way.

In his view, nobody who goes to so much trouble to get pregnant is going to have an abortion. She wanted his baby, that's the long and the short of it. She has a feeling he is right, but she also secretly wonders if this no-fault pose of his isn't also a strategy to get what *he* wants without having to take responsibility in advance. After all, he has a history of this type of thing. If only she could get him to admit to it!

He doesn't, but life picks up anyway. Now everyone is looking forward to a June arrival. At this writing, the outcome is still unknown. She still has those genetic tests to look forward to. Although she has written disparagingly about our reluctance to accept defects in offspring, she still does not feel up to that responsibility herself. So it may well turn out that she doesn't get what she wants, or gets what she thinks she doesn't want. There are still so many things that could go wrong. The only thing she does know for sure now is that she's made the right decision – even though she knows that, technically speaking, there is no such thing. Put it differently: it was the right decision for her at that time. By the time this book comes out, her fate will be known, but for the purposes of the book, it is perhaps better to leave her here, suspended in uncertainty, fearing the worst and hoping for the best, and comforted by the illusion that she has a clear idea of what she can control and what she can't.

What is the moral we ask you to draw from this story? Choose for yourself. You could say that no one is above the law when it comes to the laws of nature. Or you could say that no one is immune to the strong emotions that fertility crises arouse – that the most you can ever hope to do is develop a tiny bit of detachment, so that you can step out of the swamp of emotional turmoil from time to time and see the problem in a broader and more temperate way, and thus achieve equilibrium. You could say that every person has his or her own tortuous way of arriving at a decision, and that this one might look tortuous to an outsider, but that all's well that ends well. Or you could be the image of courtesy and refrain from passing judgement at all. You could say that you respect other people's decisions even when you don't fully understand them, that just because you don't understand them doesn't mean they don't make sense. And that none of us understand the past or can read the future well enough to know definitely whether or not a particular course of action is a mistake.

To which we reply, if there were more people like you, the world would be a much better place. But it's important to remember also – and we'll leave you with this thought – that there are problems our heroine could never solve, not even if the harshest of her judges found her behaviour to be impeccable. We have been granted the gift of reproductive choice, but as yet we don't have the bare basics that are necessary to exercise that choice properly. By these we mean the education, the autonomy, the respect, the information, and the wherewithal to carry our decisions through without obstruction. We know that a choice cannot be a choice unless there is an alternative. It is a fact there is no reproductive choice for a pregnant woman unless there is abortion. But as that battle continues, we sometimes forget to see the other end of the fertility spectrum, where the increased involvement of well-meaning professionals has meant that an individual's right to decide to *have* children is ever more in question. Which makes us ask, what are we really fighting for? Instead of saying pro-choice, shouldn't we be more specific? Shouldn't we really be saying: the right to decide if and when to have children under humane conditions – and with proper support?

APPENDIX ONE

REPRODUCTIVE HEALTH IN THE WORLD: BARE FACTS

Over 100 million acts of sexual intercourse take place each day. These result in 910,000 conceptions and 356,000 sexually transmitted bacterial and viral infections. About 50% of the conceptions are unplanned, and 25% are definitely unwanted.

About 150,000 unwanted pregnancies are terminated every day by induced abortion. One third of these abortions are performed under unsafe conditions and in adverse social and legal climates, resulting in some 500 deaths every day.

1,370 women die every day in the course of their physiological and social duty of pregnancy and childbirth, and many times more than this number have a narrow escape, though not without significant physical and psychological injuries.

Some 25,000 infants and 14,000 children aged one to four die each day. One in twelve infants born this year will not see his or her birthday, and one in eight will not see the fifth birthday.

Family planning not only prevents births, it also saves the lives of women and children. 300 million couples do not have access to family planning services.

Progress in Reproduction Research no 21 1992 WHO

APPENDIX TWO

'A user-friendly family planning service providing comprehensive advice and information is the key to ensuring better compliance,' maintains Toni Belfield, head of Information and Research at the Family Planning Association. She believes that patients have a right to full information on the advantages and disadvantages of the method they are prescribed. Any centre that offers family planning ideally should be able to:

Provide the full range of contraceptive methods, including condoms and emergency contraception.
Provide support and counselling for women requesting termination of pregnancy.
Provide counselling and referral for male and female sterilisation.
Offer pre-pregnancy planning and life style advice.
Provide pregnancy testing facilities with results available on the same day.
Give advice or refer patients for advice on sexual and relationship problems.
Provide advice on safer sex and treatment or referral for sexually transmitted diseases.
Provide well woman/man services.
Back up advice with up-to-date written materials such as family planning association leaflets.

'The way to ensure good compliance is not through telling patients what to do but giving them the choice,' concluded Mrs Belfield.

> British Journal of Sexual Medicine, May/June 1993 p 17
> Report on the Symposium 'From Menarche to Menopause'.

GLOSSARY

Abortion	The spontaneous or induced termination of a pregnancy before the fetus is viable.
Adhesion	A reaction inside the body to inflammation or infection. Fibrous tissue forms that binds internal organs in an abnormal way.
AI	*see* Artificial insemination.
AID	*see* Donor insemination.
AIH	Artificial insemination using husband's sperm.
Alzheimer's disease	A condition when the cerebral cortex of the brain shrinks resulting in dementia.
Amenorrhoea	Prolonged absence of menstruation.
Anovulatory cycles	A cycle in which ovulation does not occur.
Artificial insemination	The procedure whereby sperm is introduced into the woman's genital tract artificially instead of by natural intercourse.
Atresia	Shrinking or narrowing of a passage.
Azospermia	Total absence of sperm.
Basal body temperature	The temperature of the body taken at rest, taken immediately on waking before any activity.
BBT	*see* Basal body temperature.
Biopsy	The removal of a tiny sample of tissue from the body for investigation.
Cap	*see* Diaphragm
Cervical secretions	The secretions from the cells lining the cervix change under the influence of the sex hormones. The infertile type secretion is thick, white, sticky and flaky. It forms a barrier to sperm.

	The fertile type secretion is produced close to the time of ovulation. It gives a slippery sensation at the entrance to the vagina and resembles raw egg white. It is stretchy and transparent, its structure facilitates sperm migration.
Cervix	The narrow lower end of the uterus, containing the entrance to it. It is also called the neck of the womb.
Chlamydial infection	A sexually transmitted bacterial infection which is sometimes symptomless. It can damage the fallopian tubes causing infertility.
Chorion villus	The chorion villus is the developing placenta which grows from the same cells as the baby and therefore has the same chromosomes (inheritance factors).
Chorionic villus sampling	Chorionic villus sampling (CVS) is a test carried out after 8–10 weeks of pregnancy. It is a test for chromosomal abnormalities such as Down's syndrome. The technique involves passing a needle through the mother's abdominal wall into the uterus (a local anaesthetic is usually used to numb the skin). An ultra sound scan is done at the same time to allow the doctor to guide the needle accurately. The doctor aspirates a tiny sample of chorionic villi.
Chromosome	One of the 46 microscopic rod like structures that carry the genetic material and are present in every cell.
Cilia	Fine hair-like structures which protrude from cells lining a structure. In the case of the fallopian tube the cilia waft the egg down the tube towards the uterus.
Contraceptive pill	A pill which contains hormones. The combined pill contains the hormones oestrogen and progestogen. When taken regularly it stops ovulation. The progesterone only pill acts in a different way, it must be taken at the same time each day. The progesterone makes the cervical secretions thick and sticky which prevents the passage of sperm. It sometimes stops ovulation.
CVS	*see* Chorionic villus sampling.

Glossary

Cystic fibrosis	An inherited disease that affects the lungs of the individual.
D and C	*see* Dilatation and Curettage.
DI	*see* Donor insemination.
Diaphragm	A soft rubber device put into the vagina before intercourse to cover the cervix, and form a barrier which prevents sperm from meeting the egg. To be effective, diaphragms must be used in conjunction with a spermicidal cream, gel, foam, film or pessary. These create a contraceptive layer that keeps any sperm which may leak around the cap from passing through the cervix.
Dilatation and Curettage	This is a minor operation that involves opening the cervix with dilators and gently scraping the surface of the endometrium with an instrument called a curette. The endometrial tissue is then sent to the laboratory for analysis.
Donor insemination	Artificial insemination with donor semen.
Double Dutch method	Term used for the combination of the oral contraceptive pill and the condom. With increased awareness of HIV this is becoming a recommended method for many couples.
Egg donation	A procedure in which a woman donates her eggs to another. It is used for an infertile woman who is unable to produce her own eggs.
Ejaculation	The release of seminal fluid from the male penis at orgasm.
Embryo	The initial stages of development of the fetus from the fertilised egg to around eight weeks after conception.
Endometrium	The inner lining of the uterus which is shed during menstruation. If conception occurs the fertilised egg implants in the endometrium.
Endometriosis	The growth of endometrial tissue in areas other than the uterus e.g. the fallopian tubes or on the ovaries. It may cause infertility.
Epididymis	A tightly coiled tube within the scrotum. It connects the testes to the vas deferens. During the sperm's passage through the epididymis, they acquire the ability to move forwards by themselves.

Fallopian tubes	A pair of tubes through which the ripened ovum is transported from the ovary to the uterus. Sperm pass from the uterus to the outer third of the tube where they meet the ovum and fertilisation takes place.
Family planning	Family planning aims to enable people to choose whether and when to have a baby. This includes birth control, planning a baby, timing, conception, spacing births and infertility advice and help. Family planning embraces emotional well-being and affects the individual's enjoyment of his or her own sexuality.
Female condom	A loose and strong polyurethane tube with a ring at the top and the bottom. The upper ring is designed to cover the cervix, while the lower ring lies outside the vagina.
Femshield	*see* Female condom.
Fertilisation	The fusion of a sperm with an egg (ovum), normally in the outer third of the fallopian tube.
Fertility	The ability to produce offspring.
Fertility awareness	The awareness of the natural changes that occur in a woman during the menstrual cycle.
Fertility screening	Assessment and tests on individuals to assess their fertility status.
Fibroid	A muscular growth of tissue in the wall of the uterus. Fibroids are very common and rarely cause problems.
Fetal distress	Signs detected from the fetus which indicate that there is a problem.
Fetus	The unborn child from around eight weeks after conception till birth.
Folate	A vitamin that is essential for the normal development of a fetus. Research has shown that if a mother has not enough folate in her blood the baby may have a neural tube defect.
Follicle stimulating hormone	The hormone produced by the pituitary gland that stimulates the growth of follicles in the ovary. The growing follicles produce oestrogen and a mature ova in the largest follicle.
FSH	*see* Follicle stimulating hormone.

Glossary

Gestation	The number of weeks a woman is pregnant.
GIFT	Gamete Infra-Fallopian Transfer. This is an alternative treatment to IVF. Sperm and collected eggs are placed in the fallopian tube where fertilisation takes place.
HIV	Human Immunodeficiency Virus.
Hypercholesterolaemia	A blood cholesterol level above the normal level.
Hysterosalpingogram	An X-ray investigation which involves the injection of a small amount of fluid (that shows up with X-rays) through the cervix into the uterus. X-ray films taken show abnormalities of the uterus and blocked fallopian tubes.
Hysteroscopy	A telescope-like instrument which allows the inside of the uterus to be inspected under direct vision.
Implantation	The process by which the fertilised egg implants into the endometrium.
In-vitro fertilisation	This involves removing one or more mature eggs from the ovary, fertilising the eggs outside the body with sperm. Then transferring one or more of the fertilised eggs back into the uterus.
Intra uterine device	This is a small plastic device, which may or may not also bear a chemical such as copper or contain a hormone. It is inserted into the uterus by a doctor. It works mainly by preventing the egg and sperm meeting; or it may delay the egg coming down the fallopian tube, or prevent an egg from implanting into the uterus.
IUCD	Intra uterine Contraceptive Device
IUD	*see* Intra uterine device.
IUI	Intra uterine insemination
IVF	*see* In-vitro fertilisation.
Lactational amenorrhoea method	If a mother is fully breast-feeding and her baby is less than six months old, so long as her periods have not returned research has shown that 98 per cent are protected from pregnancy.
Laparoscopy & Dye	This is a surgical procedure used to investigate the pelvis. It involves a telescope-like instrument called a laparoscope being inserted

into the abdominal cavity through a tiny incision. The laparoscope is attached to a tiny light source. By looking through the laparoscope the gynaecologist can see abnormalities such as endometriosis or ovarian cysts. If there is a suspected blockage in the fallopian tubes a dye is flushed through the tubes from the uterus. If the dye is seen coming through it means the fallopian tube is not blocked.

LH *see* Luteinising hormone.

Listeriosis An illness caused by a bacteria called Listeria monocytogenes. Listeriosis is a mild flu-like illness which can result in miscarriage, still birth, or severe illness in the newborn baby.

Luteal phase *see* Post ovulatory phase.

Luteinising hormone The hormone produced by the pituitary that causes the egg to be released from the follicle on the ovary. It also stimulates the development and maintenance of the corpus luteum.

Menarche The age at which menstruation begins.

Menopause The permanent cessation of menstruation due to failure of ovulation and hormone production by the ovaries.

Menstruation The cyclical period of bleeding from the uterus as the endometrium is shed.

Micro manipulation In cases of male infertility the ability of the sperm to penetrate the outer coating of the egg is assisted by making a tiny hole in the outer coating in order to allow sperm to penetrate. A micro manipulator is used which magnifies the egg and allows intricate procedures to be performed.

Miscarriage The spontaneous ending of a pregnancy before the fetus is viable.

Missed abortion When during a pregnancy the fetus has died but a woman has not had a bleed.

Mittelschmertz pain A pain some women experience on one side of the lower abdomen at the time of ovulation.

Natural family planning (NFP) Methods for planning or preventing pregnancy by observation of the naturally occurring signs and symptoms of the fertile and infertile phases of the menstrual cycle (WHO definition).

Glossary

	If a couple choose to use barrier methods during the fertile phase this is referred to as fertility awareness with barriers and not natural family planning.
Neural tube defect	An abnormality during development of the fetus of the brain or the spinal chord, e.g. spina bifida, anencephaly or hydrocephalus.
Oestrogen	A hormone produced mainly by the ovaries, responsible for the development of the female secondary sex characteristics, and control of the menstrual cycle. Increasing oestrogen levels in the first part of the menstrual cycle produce changes in the cervix and the cervical secretions which indicate fertility.
Oligosperma	Too few sperm.
Ovary	One of a pair of female sex organs (ovaries) which produce ova and the female sex hormones oestrogen and progesterone.
Ovum	The mature female sex cell or egg.
Ovum donation	*see* Egg donation.
Pill	*see* Contraceptive pill.
Pituitary gland	The 'master gland' at the base of the brain which produces many important hormones, some of which trigger other glands into making their own hormones. The pituitary functions include hormonal control of the sex glands.
Placenta praevia	When the placenta is partially or completely lying over the cervix it is called a placenta praevia. When this occurs the baby cannot be delivered via the vagina without the mother being at grave risk of a serious haemorrhage. She therefore must have a Caesarean section.
Post Ovulatory phase	The phase from ovulation to the onset of the next menstruation.
Pre-conceptual care	Also known as pre-pregnancy screening: information and investigations that are offered to couples planning a baby.
Pre-embryo	The fertilised egg in its earliest stage of development. At present this term is used to describe a fertilised egg during the first two weeks of life before the streak of tissue that

Pre-ovulatory phase	The phase from the beginning of menstruation till ovulation.
Progesterone	A hormone produced after ovulation by the corpus luteum on the ovary. It prepares the endometrium for a possible pregnancy. It is also responsible for the rise in basal body temperature, and for the cervical secretions to change to being thick and sticky.
Progestogen	Progesterone is one of a class of substances known as progestogens. Many different ones have been synthesised and are used in the oral contraceptive pills.
Prolactin	A pituitary hormone which stimulates the production of breast milk and inhibits the ovarian production of oestrogen.
Scrotum	The pouch of skin containing the testes.
Semen	*see* Seminal fluid.
Seminal fluid	The fluid ejaculated from the penis at orgasm. The fluid contains sperm and secretions from the seminal vesicles and prostate gland.
Seminal vesicles	A pair of sacs which open into the top of the male urethra. Its secretions form part of the seminal fluid.
Sperm	The mature male sex cell.
Spermatozoon (plural Spermatozoa)	*see* Sperm.
Spina bifida	An abnormality of the development of the spine and in more serious cases the spinal chord resulting in the nerves being damaged and the individual being paralysed.
Sponge (contraceptive)	A female barrier method of contraception. The sponge is impregnated with a spermicidal. It is inserted into the vagina covering the cervix.
Spinnbarkeit test	A test done on cervical secretions to assess height to which it can be stretched.
Sterilisation	An operation done to a man or woman that renders him or her permanently infertile. It may be reversed in some cases. *See* Tubal ligation.

Glossary

Stillbirth When a baby dies before it is born.

Stress cycles Abnormalities of the menstrual cycle caused by either mental or physical stress.

Temperature method of family planning A method of natural family planning which involves taking your temperature on waking. The post-ovulatory infertile phase is identified by a sustained rise in the basal body temperature.

Testicle One of a pair of male sex organs which produces sperm and the male sex hormones called androgens one of which is testosterone.

Testis (plural Testes) *see* Testicle.

Testosterone A hormone produced by the testes, responsible for the development of male secondary sex characteristics and functioning of the male reproductive organs. Small amounts of testosterone are produced in women.

Toxoplasmosis A mild flu-like illness caused by a parasite called Toxoplasma gondii. It is found in raw meat, unpasteurised goat's milk or unpasteurised goat's milk products, unwashed, uncooked fruit and vegetables and cat faeces. Toxoplasmosis infection in the fetus can cause problems with the eye sight and hydrocephalus which might cause brain damage.

Tubal Ligation A surgical operation used to sterilise women. The fallopian tubes are cut and the fallopian tubes are closed so the egg cannot travel down them to meet the sperm.

Ultrasound A method of examining the internal organs of the body using high frequency sound waves. The images the sound waves provide look very similar to X-rays but they have great advantages, unlike X-rays they do not damage the body tissue.

Undescended Testis When the testis has not descended to the scrotum. It may lie above the scrotum or in the abdominal cavity. An undescended testis may not function normally. Male infertility is sometimes because of both testes being undescended.

Urethra	The tube that conveys urine from the bladder to outside the body.
Uterus	The pear-shaped muscular organ whose lining is called the endometrium in which the fertilised egg implants. The muscular contractions of the uterus push the infant out through the birth canal at the time of birth. If implantation does not take place the uterine linings shed at menstruation.
Vagina	The muscular canal extending from the cervix to the opening at the vulva. Sperm are deposited in the vagina during intercourse. It is also through this canal that the baby is delivered.
Vaginal prolapse	When the vaginal wall is lax and protrudes beyond the entrance of the vagina.
Vaginismus	A spasm of the muscles of the vagina that occurs whenever intercourse is attempted.
Vas deferens	One of a pair of tubes which convey the seminal fluid from the testis to the urethra.
Vasectomy	An operation done to sterilise a male. The vas deferens on each side is cut and the ends separated to prevent sperm travelling from the testes to the urethra.
Wedge resection of the ovary	An abdominal operation which involves removing a wedge section of the ovary. The cut edges are sewn back together again. It is used to treat polycystic ovary syndrome.
Womb	*see* Uterus.
Womb rejuvenation	The treatment offered to a woman who has reached the menopause and wishes to have a baby. She is given hormones that prepare the uterus for IVF.

NOTES

See bibliography for full publication details of references

TWO
1. Guillebaud, *The Pill* p 23

FIVE
1. Haste, *Rules of Desire*, p 206
2. General Household Survey 1991

SIX
1. FPA factsheet, July 1992, p 1

SEVEN
1. Anon, 'Abortion, a Conflict', *Observer*

NINE
1. Kitzinger, Sheila, *Ourselves as Mothers* p 40

TWELVE
1. Jennings, 'A Lifeline Offering Support . . .' p 95
2. Ellmann, *Thinking About Women*, pp 177–182
3. Luker, *Taking Chances*, p 16
4. ibid. p 28
5. ibid. p 34
6. ibid. p 64
7. ibid. p 64
8. ibid. p 35
9. ibid. p 67
10. ibid. p 36

11. ibid. p 67
12. ibid. p 8
13. Miller, Warren B, 'Psychological Vulnerability . . .' pp 199–201
14. ibid., 'Why Some Women . . .' p 30
15. ibid.
16. Boyle, Mary, 'Contraception and Abortion', *Pregnancy, Contraception and Family Planning Services in Industrialised Countries* (ed. Elise Jones), p 157
17. ibid.
18. ibid.
19. Luker, *Taking Chances*, p 59

THIRTEEN
1. Kitzinger, *Ourselves as Mothers*, p 35
2. Anderson, *Approaches to the History . . .*, p 18
3. ibid. p 20
4. ibid. pp 39–64
5. ibid. p 69
6. Donzelot, *The Policing of Families*, p 25
7. ibid. p 181
8. Stopes *Wise Parenthood*, dedication page
9. ibid. pp 1–2
10. ibid. p 9
11. ibid. pp 17–19
12. ibid. p 21
13. ibid. p 27
14. ibid. p 44
15. Fisher, William, Adolescents, Sex and Contraception, 'Adolescent Contraception: Summary and Recommendations', p 273

FOURTEEN
1. Evans-Pritchard, Ambrose, *Sunday Telegraph* 1 March 1993
2. ibid.
3. Reilly, Helen, *GP News*

FIFTEEN
1. Faludi, *Backlash*, p 49
2. Tan, *Infertility: Your Questions Answered* p 4
3. ibid.
4. Ellmann, *Thinking About Women* pp 13–14

SIXTEEN
1. Belfield, Toni, article in Contraception, Reed Healthcare, 1991 p 6
2. Guillebaud, *The Pill*, p 21

Notes

3. ibid. p 126 see also Vessey, Prof. Martin, et al, 'Return of Fertility Post-Pill', Oxford FPA Study in *British Journal of Family Planning*, 1986 vol. 11 pp 120–40
4. ibid. p 181
5. ibid. p 208
6. ibid. p 208
7. ibid. p 218
8. ibid. p 218
9. Mosse, *The Fertility and Contraception Book*, pp 164–195
10. Guillebaud, *The Pill* p 232
11. Mosse, *The Fertility and Contraception Book*, p 186
12. ibid.
13. Kishen, article in Contraception, Reed Healthcare, pp 28–35
14. Guillebaud, *The Pill*, p 252
15. Dr E. Clubb, Dr C. Pyper and Jane Knight: Pilot Study on cost effectiveness of teaching fertility awareness in general practice 1991
16. Wade 1979 USA Sympto-thermal/ovulation method comparative study.
17. Flynn, Anne Marie, FCOG Update, pp 151–158
18. Mosse, *The Fertility and Contraception Book*, p 303
19. ibid. p 302
20. Ibid. p 305
21. ibid.
22. Guillebaud, *The Pill*, pp 253–254
23. Mosse, *The Fertility and Contraception Book*, p 315
24. ibid. p 326
25. Illmann, 'Why Sisters Are . . .' *Guardian*
26. GP Abortion, Haymarket Publications, pp 43–48
27. 'Genetic Services . . . A Guide'
28. ibid.
29. 'Before You Conceive' Expert Advice from the Royal College of Midwives leaflet
30. McKie, 'Sex Selection . . .', *Observer*
31. Thistle, 'Premature Baby Care . . .' p 19
32. *Drug and Therapeutics Bulletin*, Vol 32, No 3
33. McCauley A.P., Geller J.A., *Decisions for Norplant Programs Population Reports*. Series K, No 4. Baltimore: Johns Hopkins University Population Information Program, November 1992
34. Sivin I. International experience with Norplant and Norplant-2 contraceptives, *Stud Fam Plann* 1988; 19: 81–94
35. Shoupe D., Mishell D.R. Jr, Bopp B.L., Fielding M., 'The significance of bleeding patterns in Norplant implant users', *Obstet Gynecol* 1991; 77:256

SEVENTEEN

1. Faludi, *Backlash*, p 50
2. Winston, Prof., 'Infertility . . .' pp 16–17
3. Winn, 'The Fertile Mind', p 95
4. WHO Progress Newsletter pp 4–5
5. Tan, *Infertility* . . . p 97
6. Tan, *Infertility*, IVF Success Rate Charts, pp 120–122
7. Winston, Prof. Robert, Symposium on Sex Hormones and General Practice, Regents College, London Dec 1992
8. Office of Population Censuses and Surveys Birth Statistics 1990
9. Leridon, 'Patterns of fertility . . .', *Biosoc Sci Supplement*
10. Sauer, 'Pregnancy After Age Fifty . . .', *Lancet* pp 321–323
11. Winston, Prof., *Well Woman Team*, issue 11 1993
12. 'Assisted Pregnancy at 62 may force age limit', Interview with Ian Craft, *GP Magazine*, 1 May 1993

BIBLIOGRAPHY

BOOKS

Anderson, Michael, *Approaches to the History of the Western Family 1500–1914*, Macmillan, London, 1980

Byrne, Donn, Fisher, Williams, et al., *Adolescents, Sex and Contraception*, Laurence Erlbaum Associations, Hillsdale, New Jersey and London 1983

Clubb, Dr Elizabeth and Knight, Jane, *Fertility: A Comprehensive Guide to Natural Family Planning*, David and Charles, London, 1992 edition

Donzelot, Jacques, *The Policing of Families*, Hutchinson, London, 1980

Ellmann, Mary, *Thinking About Women*, Virago, London, 1969

Faludi, Susan, *Backlash: The Undeclared War Against Women*, Chatto and Windus, London, 1992

Fox, G. L., *The Childbearing Decision: Fertility Attitudes and Behaviour*, Sage, London 1992

Gerson, Kathleen, *Hard Choices: How Women Decide About Work, Career and Motherhood*, University of California Press, Berkeley/London 1985

Greer, Germaine, *Sex and Destiny – the Politics of Human Fertility*, Secker and Warburg, 1984

Guillebaud, John, *The Pill*, Oxford University Press, Oxford 1991

Haste, Cate, *Rules of Desire: Sex in Britain, World War I to the Present*, Chatto and Windus, London 1992

Jones, Elise (Jacqueline Darroch Forest, Stanley K. Henshaw, Jane Silverman and Aida Torres) *Pregnancy, Contraception and Family Planning Services in Industrialised Countries*, Yale, New Haven, 1989.

Kaplan, Pat, *The Cultural Construction of Sexuality*, Tavistock Routledge, London 1987

Kitzinger, Sheila, *Ourselves as Mothers*, Doubleday, London 1992

Kitzinger, Sheila, *Woman's Experience of Sex*, Dorling Kindersley, London 1983

Klein, Debby, and Kaufman, Tara, *Unwanted Pregnancy*, Penguin, London 1992

Luker, Kristin, *Taking Chances: Abortion and the Decision Not to Contracept*, University of California Press, Berkeley, 1975

McPherson, Ann (ed), *Women's Problems in General Practice*, Oxford University Press, Oxford, 1992 edition

McNeil, Maureen (ed) et al, *New Reproductive Technologies*, Macmillan, London, 1990

Martin, Emily, *The Woman in the Body*, Open University Press, Buckingham 1989

Mosse, Julia, and Heaton, Josephine, *The Fertility and Contraception Book*, Faber, London 1990

Neuberger, Julia, *Whatever's Happening to Women?*, Kyle Cathie, London 1991

Oakley, Ann, *Sex, Gender and Society*, New Society/Gower, London, 1989 edition

Orbach, Suzie, and Eichenbaum, Luise, *Understanding Women*, Penguin, London 1983

Ramphal, Sridath, *Our Country, the Planet*, Lime Tree, London 1992

Shorter, Edward, *The Making of the Modern Family*, Fontana, London 1979

Stanworth, Michelle, *Reproductive Technologies: Gender, Motherhood and Medicine*, Blackwell, Oxford 1987

Stopes, Marie, *Wise Parenthood*, GP Putnam's Sons, London 1923

Tan, S. I., and Jacobs, H. S., *Infertility: Your Questions Answered*, McGraw Hill, London 1991

Yates, Frank, *Risk-Taking Behavior*, University of Michigan, Ann Arbor, Michigan, John Wiley and Sons 1992

ARTICLES AND SUPPLEMENTS

Cameron, Iain T, 'Unwanted Pregnancy', *Postgraduate Update*, 15 Dec 1991

Coglan, Andy, 'Immune to Pregnancy?' *New Scientist*, 17 Oct 1992

Eisen, Marvin et al, 'Evaluating the Impact of a Theory-Based Sexuality and Contraceptive Education Program', *Family Planning Perspectives*, Vol 22 No 6 Nov/Dec 1990, pp 261–71

Bibliography

Evans-Pritchard, Ambrose, 'Ghetto school where all the girls bring their babies too', *Sunday Telegraph*, 31 Jan 1993

Flynn, Anne Marie, 'Natural Methods of Fertility Control', *FCOG Update*, Jul 1991 pp 39–43 and Aug 1991 pp 151–8

Forrest, Jacqueline Darroch, 'The Delivery of Family Planning Services in the United States', *Family Planning Perspectives*, Vol 20 No 2 Mar/Apr 1988, pp 88–95

Hadlington, Simon, 'Drug Offers Hope in Male Sterility', *Doctor*, 18 Apr 1991

Haslam, David, 'Where Have All Those Sperm Gone?' World Of Medicine, *GP*, 2 Oct 1992

Hull, Prof. Michael, 'Infertility Needs and Effectiveness' Report from the University of Bristol, Serone Laboratories UK Ltd 1992

Illman, John, 'Why Sisters Are Doing It for Themselves', *Guardian*, 3 Nov 1992

Jennings, Sue, 'A Lifeline Offering Support: Nurses' Role in Fertility Counselling', *Professional Nurse*, May 1992

Jones, Elise F, 'Unintended Pregnancy, Contraceptive Practice and Family Planning Services in Developed Countries', *Family Planning Perspectives*, Vol 20 No 2 Mar/Apr 1988, pp 53–67

Kirby, Douglas, 'Reducing the Risk: Impact of a New Curriculum on Sexual Risk-Taking', *Family Planning Perspectives*, Vol 23, No 6, Nov/Dec 1991, pp 253–5

Kishen, Dr Meera, 'Barrier Methods, Natural Family Planning and Sterilisation, Contraception', *Reed Healthcare Communications*, London, 1991

Klitsch, Michael, 'Antiprogestins and the Abortion Controversy: A Progress Report', *Family Planning Perspectives*, Vol 23 No 6 Nov/Dec 1991 pp 275–282

Kost, Kathryn et al, 'Comparing the Health Risks and Benefits of Contraceptive Choices', *Family Planning Perspectives*, Vol 23 No 2, Mar/Apr 1991, p 54

Leridon, J. H., 'Patterns of fertility at later ages of reproduction', *Biosoc Sci Supplement* Vol 6 1979, pp 59–64

Lundberg, Shelly, 'Effects of State Welfare, Abortion and Family Planning Policies on Premarital Childbearing Among White Adolescents', *Family Planning Perspectives*, Vol 23 No 6 Nov/Dec 1991, p 246

McKie, Robin, 'Sex Selection Clinic "A Waste of Money" ' *Observer* 31 Jan 1993

Miller, Susan Katz, 'Warning: Smoking May Damage Your Sperm', *New Scientist*, 17 Oct 1992

Miller, Warren B, 'Why Some Women Fail to Use Their Contraceptive Method: A Psychological Investigation', *Family Planning Perspectives*, Vol 18 No 1 Jan/Feb 1986, pp 27–32

Miller, Warren B, 'Psychological Vulnerability to Unwanted Pregnancy', ibid. Vol 5 No 4, 1973, pp 199–201

Moore, Suzanne, 'Unwanted Pain of an Unwanted Pregnancy', *Guardian* 8 Oct 1992, p 32

Moore, Thomas, 'New Hope for Impotence', *GP*, 15 Mar 1991

Reilly, Helen, 'Doctors Promise "Perfect" Children' *GP News* 'Assisted pregnancy at 62 may force age limit', *GP News*, 1 May 1992: Interview with Prof. Ian Craft

Rind, Patricia, 'Peer Support to Keep Teenagers Alive and Well', *Family Planning Perspectives*, Vol 24 No 1 Jan/Feb 1992, p 36

Ross, John A, 'Contraception: Short-Term vs Long-Term Failure Rates', *Family Planning Perspectives*, Vol 21 No 6 Nov/Dec 1989 pp 275–277

Sauer, M. V. Paulson, R. J. Lobo Ra, 'Pregnancy After Age Fifty: application of oocyte donation after the natural menopause', *Lancet* Vol 341 1993, pp 321–323

Silverman, Jane et al, 'The Delivery of Family Planning and Health Services in Great Britain', *Family Planning Perspectives*, Vol 20 No 2 Mar/Apr 1988, pp 68–74

Storm, Rachel, 'The Fertile Effects of Drama Used to Help the Childless', *Observer* 12 Oct 1988

Sudlow, C. L. M., Margaret Jackson Memorial Prize Essay, 'The Contraceptive Effect of Breastfeeding', *British Journal of Family Planning*, Vol 17 1991, pp 56–59

Thistle, Dr Jill, 'Premature Baby Care Needs New Legal Limits', *Mimms Magazine Weekly*, 23 Mar 1993

Winn, Denise, 'The Fertile Mind', *GH*, Feb 1988

Wineberg, Howard, 'Variations in Fertility by Marital Status and Marriage Order', *Family Planning Perspectives*, Vol 23 No 6 Nov/Dec 1991, p 256

Winston, Prof., *Well Woman Team*, issue 11 1993

Winston, Prof., R. M. L., et al, 'Infertility, Update Postgraduate Centre Series', *Reed Healthcare Communications*, London 1991

Winter, Laraine, 'The Role of Sexual Self-Concept in the Use of Contraceptives', *Family Planning Perspectives*, Vol 20 No 3 May/Jun 1988, pp 123–27

Bibliography

UNATTRIBUTED ARTICLES AND BROCHURES

'Abortion', GP Top 100
'Abortion', *Guardian* Education, 27 Oct 1992
'Abortion, A Conflict that Can Never Be Resolved', Anon. *Observer* Colour Supplement, 13 Nov 1988
'Before You Conceive: Expert Advice from the Royal College of Midwives' (leaflet)
Family Planning Association Factsheet, 'Contraception: Attitudes and Practice', Jul 1992
Family Planning Association Factsheet, 'Contraceptive Usage and Trends in the United Kingdom', Aug 1992
'Fertility Objectives', United States Department of Health and Human Services
'Genetic Services, Prenatal Diagnosis and Pregnancy Screening in the Oxford Region: A Guide', Department of Medical Genetics, Churchill Hospital, Oxford 10 Jan 1991
General Household Survey 1991
'No Regrets', British Organisation of Non-Parents pamphlet
Office of Population Census and Surveys and Birth Statistics 1990 series FMI No 19, London HMSO 1991
WHO Progress Newsletter of the Special Programme of Reproductive Development and Research Training in Human Reproduction No 15 1990 pp 4–5

VIDEO

'Fertility, A Guide to Natural Family Planning', produced by Dr E. Clubb and Jane Knight, Dept of Medical Illustration, John Radcliffe Hospital, University of Oxford, Oxford OX3 9DU

USEFUL ADDRESSES

Medical Organisations

National Association of Family Planning Doctors
27 Sussex Place
Regent's Park
London NW1 4RG
Tel: 071 724 2441

Brook Advisory Centres (Head Office)
153a East Street
London SE17 2SD
Tel: 071 708 1234

British Pregnancy Advisory Service (BPAS)
1st floor Guildhall Building
Navigation Street
Birmingham B2 4BT
Tel: 021 643 1461

National Childbirth Trust
Alexandra House
Oldham Terrace
London W3 6NH
Tel: 081 992 8637

Women's Health Concern
PO Box 1629
London W8 6AU
Tel: 071 938 3932

Useful Addresses

Institute of Psychosexual Medicine
11 Chandos Street
London W1M 9DE
Tel: 071 580 0631

Women's Health (formerly WHRRIC)
52 Featherstone Street
London EC1Y 8RT
Tel: 071 251 6333

Family Planning

Family Planning Association
& Family Planning Information Service
27–35 Mortimer Street
London W1N 7RJ
Tel: 071 636 7866

National Natural Family Planning Service
1 Blythe Mews
Blythe Road
London W14 0NW
Tel: 071 371 1341

National Association Natural Family Planning Teachers
NFPO Centre
Birmingham B15 2TG
Tel: 021 472 1377 (Ext 4219)

Counselling

British Association of Counsellors
37a Sheep Street
Rugby CV21 3BX
Tel: 0788 578328

Catholic Marriage Advisory Council
Clitherow House
1 Blythe Mews
Blythe Road
London W14 0NW
Tel: 071 371 1341

Relate
National Marriage Guidance
Herbert Gray College
Little Church Street
Rugby CV21 3AP
Tel: 0788 573241

Tavistock Centre
120 Belsize Lane
London NW3 5BA
Tel: 071 435 7111

Childbirth and Breast-feeding

Birthright
27 Sussex Place
Regents Park
London NW1 4SP
Tel: 071 262 5337

La Leche League
BM 2434
London WC1N 3XX
Tel: 071 242 1278

The National Childbirth Trust
Alexandra House
Oldham Terrace
Acton
London W3 6NH
Tel: 081 992 8637

Infertility

Issue (the National Fertility Association)
509 Aldridge Road
Great Barr
Birmingham B44 8NA
Tel: 021 344 4414

British Pregnancy Advisory Service (BPAS)
1st floor Guildhall Building

Useful Addresses

Navigation Street
Birmingham B2 4BT
Tel: 021 643 1461

Child
Suite 219 Caledonian House
98 The Centre
Feltham
Middlesex TW13 4BH
Tel: 081 893 7110

Gynaecological/Obstetrics

Women's Nutritional Advisory Service
PO Box 268
Lewis
East Sussex BN7 2QN
Tel: 0273 487366

Miscarriage Association
c/o Clayton Hospital
Northgate
Wakefield
West Yorkshire WF1 3JS
Tel: 092 420 0799

Pelvic Inflammatory Disease Group
Womens Health
52 Featherstone Street
London EC1Y 8RT
Tel: 071 251 6580

Pregnancy Counselling

British Pregnancy Advisory Service (BPAS)
1st floor Guildhall Building
Navigation Street
Birmingham B2 4BT
Tel: 021 643 1461

Life Headquarters
1a Newbold Terrace

Leamington Spa
Warwickshire
CV32 4EA
Tel: 0926 421 587

Brook Advisory Centres (Head Office)
153a East Street
London SE17 2SD
Tel: 071 708 1234

Pro Choice Alliance
27–35 Mortimer Street
London W1N 7RJ
Tel: 071 636 4619

Pre-conceptual Care

Foresight
28 The Paddock
Godalming
Surrey GU7 1XD
Tel: 0483 427 839

The Toxoplasmosis Trust
67–71 Collier Street
London N1 9BE
Tel: 071 713 0663
Helpline 071 713 0599

Listeria Support Group
Worlingworth
Woodbridge
Suffolk IP13 7NZ
Tel: 0728 628287

HIV/AIDS

Terrence Higgins Trust
52–54 Grays Inn Road
London WC1X 8JU
Tel: 071 831 0330
Helpline 071 242 1010

Useful Addresses

Positively Women
5 Sebastian Street
London EC1 V0HE
Tel: 071 490 5515
Helpline 071 490 2327

National AIDS Helpline
Tel: 0800 567123

Support Network

The Stillbirth and Neonatal Death Society (SANDS)
28 Portland Place
London W1N 4DE
Tel: 071 436 5881

The Miscarriage Association (MA)
Clayton Hospital
Northgate Wakefield
West Yorks WF1 3SJ
Tel: 0924 200799

Nippers Bereavement Group
c/o Sam Segal Perinatal Unit
St Mary's Hospital
Praed Street
London W2 1NY
Tel: 071 725 1487

Support Around Termination for Abnormality (SAFTA)
29–30 Soho Square
London W1V 6JB
Tel: 071 439 6124

Health Promotion Agencies

The Health Education Authority
Hamilton House
Mabledon Place
London WC1H 9TX
Tel: 071 383 3833

Adoption

British Agency for Adoption and Fostering (BAAF)
11 Southwark Street
London SE1
Tel: 071 407 8800

Catholic Adoption
The Catholic Children's Society
73 St Charles Square
London W10 6EJ
Tel: 081 969 5305

Domestic Violence

Women's Aid Federation
PO Box 391
Bristol BS99 7WS
Tel: 0272 633494

Rape Crisis Centre
PO Box 69
London WC1X 9NJ
Tel: 071 837 1600

Eating Disorders

Women's Therapy Centre
6–9 Manor Gardens
London N7 6LA
Tel: 071 263 6200

Individuals with Special Needs

Association for Spina Bifida and Hydrocephalus (ASBAH)
123 East Barnet
New Barnet
Herts EN4 8RF
Tel: 081 449 0475

Cleft Lip and Palate Organisation (CLAPA)
Dental Department

Useful Addresses

Hospital for Sick Children
Great Ormond Street
London WC1N 3JH
Tel: 071 829 8614

Cystic Fibrosis Research
Alexandra House
5 Blythe Road
Bromley
Kent BR1 3RS
Tel: 081 464 7211

Disabled Living Foundation
380–384 Harrow Road
London W9 2HU
Tel: 071 289 6111

Down's Syndrome Association (DSA)
155 Mitcham Road
London SW1 9PG
Tel: 081 682 4001

Haemophilia Society
123 Westminster Bridge Road
London SE1 7HR
Tel: 071 928 2020

Royal Society for Mentally Handicapped Children and Adults
123 Golden Lane
London EC1Y 0RT
Tel: 071 454 0454

Muscular Dystrophy Group
7–11 Prescott Place
London SW4 6BS
Tel: 071 720 8055

National Deaf Children's Society
45 Hereford Road
London W2 5AH
Tel: 071 229 9272

...st for Metabolic Diseases in Children (RTMDC)
...et
Nantwich
Cheshire CW5 5NF
Tel: 0270 250221

Royal Institute for the Blind
224 Great Portland Street
London W1N 6AA
Tel: 071 388 1266

National Deaf Blind and Rubella Association (SENSE)
11–13 Clifton Terrace
Finsbury Park
London N4 3SR
Tel: 071 272 7774

Sickle Cell Society
54 Station Road
Harlesden
London NW10 4UA
Tel: 081 961 7795/8346

One Parent Families

National Council for One Parent Families
255 Kentish Town Road
London NW5 2LX
Tel: 071 267 1361

Gingerbread
35 Wellington Street
London WC2E 7BN
Tel: 071 240 0953

INDEX

The alphabetical glossary on pages 241–9 should also be consulted

Abortion
   attitude later 6; case studies 55–9, 61–4, 64–6, 66–7, 67–8, 70–3, 74; 'do-it-yourself' (menstrual extraction) 191; illegal 107–8; legal 124–5, 192–3; as let-out clause 100; natural 84–5; percentage of pregnancies terminated 54; support services 54–74; trauma 59–61; unwanted pregnancy 193–5; views on 44, 49, 150; for wanted pregnancy 195–200; woman's decision? 99–100
Abortion pill 125
Abstinence from sex, problems 187
Acupuncture 213
Adoption 10, 97
Adoptive parents 10, 20
   case study 143–4
AIDS 180, 182
   and AID 226
Alcohol and pregnancy 201, 202
Alpha Fetoprotein (AFP) test 197–8
Ambivalence towards pregnancy 39, 100, 121
Amniocentesis 97, 105, 147, 193, 199
Anencephaly, tests for 198
Anxiety *see* Stress
Artificial insemination 217

husband's semen (AIH) 225–6; by other donor (AID) 226
Assisted conception 225
see also GIFT; IVF
Atresia 156

Babies, premature 208–10
Barrier method of contraception 178–82
Basal Body Temperature charts *see* Temperature charts
Belfield, Toni 168, 240
Billings method of FP 186
Biological clock 153
Bioself device in natural FP 185
Birth control *see* Contraception
Boyce, Mary 117–18
Breast-feeding as birth control 188
British Organisation of Non-Parents, questions 138–40
Broodiness 18–19, 32, 33, 98

Cancer and contraceptives 171, 172, 174, 179
Caps (barrier method) 38, 178–81
Cervical cap 178, 179, 180
Cervical secretions 155, 159, 160, 161–2, 175, 216, 218
   patterns noted in natural FP 184, 185
Cervix 160–1, 162, 178, 179–81

changes noted in natural FP 184, 185;
problems with 216
Chard, Timothy 148
Chemotherapy and pregnancy 204
Children
 imaginary 95, 101, 120; 'perfect' and
 'superior' 148–9; the reality 97–8;
 spacing of childbearing 129;
 unwanted, social problems of 11
Chlamidia 211
Chorionic villus sampling (CVS) 147,
 197
Cilia 158
Clomiphene drug 173, 214, 221
Combined contraceptive pill 170–3
Condoms 36, 37, 180–1
 female 38, 180; use with pill 171–2;
 safety rate 182
Cone biopsies 216
Contraception 35–42
 choice based on body knowledge 163;
 drudgery to women 99; and fertility
 166–7; history 128–9; ignorance of
 115; partial use 5–6, 33, 114, 116–
 17; research 173; and sex education
 136; 'women's business' 35–6
'Contraceptive mentality' 166
Contraceptives
 basis of choice 168; emergency 191–3;
 list of types 167; *see also under
 individual types*
Craft, Prof. Ian 229
Cystic fibrosis, tests for 147

Danazol drug 215–16
Defects in fetuses, screening for 147–8
Depo-provera drug 176
Diaphragm method of contraception
 178, 179, 180
Diet during pregnancy 201, 203–4
Dilatation and curettage (D and C)
 219–20
Doctors 93, 103–8
 conspiracy with mothers 131–2, 134–
 5; helpful 109–11; and parents'
 decisions 7; four utopian types
 127–8
Donzelot, Jacques 131–2, 134
Double Dutch method of contraception
 172
Down's syndrome children 105, 122,
 147
 risk table 196; tests for 197, 198–9
Drinking alcohol during pregnancy 201,
 202
Drug addiction and pregnancy 202

Ectopic pregnancies 158, 175, 184, 190,
 214
Eggs
 fertilisation 158–9; production 154,
 156; release 158, 163–4
Ejaculation 157
Ellmann, Mary 112, 163–4
Emergency contraception 191–3
Endometriosis 215–16, 219
Endoscopy 219
Entwhistle, Paul 213
Ethics *see* Moral aspects
Eugenics 131–3, 148

Fallopian tubes 158, 159
 problems 214, 219, 221
Faludi, Susan 154, 211
Families 129–30
 the reality 24–5
Family planning xi, 9, 131–2
 see also Contraception
Family Planning Act 1967 107
Family Research Council 147
Female barrier methods of contraception
 178–81
Female *see also* Women
Feminists
 and choice 54; and motherhood 20
Femring 178
Fertilisation in fallopian tube 158–9
 timing 159
Fertility
 care for 200–6; conception rate 211;
 controllability of 11–13; course of

Index

155; four classic fertility utopians 127–8; lack of knowledge xi, 4–5, 81; politics of 5, 127–41; problems and help-seeking 217–18; research 169–70; statistics on 169–70; studies of over-40s 212; suppression of 136

Fertility awareness 163, 186, 187–8, 234–5
Fertility control 150–1, 165–210
  decision making 204–10
Fertility rate 153–4
Fertility treatment 93–4, 146
Fetus, a baby after 24 weeks 208
Fibroids 215, 219
Folate deficiency 201–2

Gender selection 207–8
  clinics 146
Genetic screening 5, 124, 125, 147, 151, 212
Genetics *see also* Eugenics
GIFT (gamete intra-fallopian transfer) 87, 90, 225
Glover, Jonathan 208
Gratification, childbearing as 16
Guillebaud, John 9, 169, 172, 173, 174, 190

Haste, Cate 36
Heart disease, and the pill 171, 172, 174
Herbal remedies, and pregnancy 202
HIV virus 165, 171, 180, 181
  and pregnancy 203
Hormones 156, 157, 158, 160, 170, 171
  deficiency in men 220, 221; deficiency in women 221
Human Fertilisation and Embryology Authority (HFEA) 229
Hypnotherapy 213
Hysteroscopy 219
Hysterosalpingogram 219

Illnesses and pregnancy 202–3
Implantation 125
Impotence in men 156, 217
Impulsive behaviour 204

In vitro fertilisation (IVF) 10, 11, 87, 146, 217, 222, 223–5, 226–7
Incompleteness, women's feeling 91, 92
Infertility
  causes, in over-40s 212; feelings on discovery 7; male 86, 156, 220; miseries of 81–95; physical problems 214–27; problems 212–13; shame factor 84–6, 87, 91, 92
'Infertility epidemic' 153
Injectable progestogen 175–7
Inter-uterine devices (IUDs) 38, 162, 182–4
  containing progestogen 177–8; insertion after intercourse 192
Intercourse, timing 218
Interview technique of this study xii–xiii
Intra-cervical device 177
Intuition, praised 120–1

Kitzinger, Sheila 93

Laparoscopy 215, 219
Legitimacy and illegitimacy 44, 226
Lesbian parents 32, 93–4, 226
Listeriosis 203
Liver (food) and pregnancy 201
London Fertility and Gynaecology Centre 229
London Gender Clinic 207
Lubricants for intercourse 182
Luker, Kristin 113, 115–16, 118

Male *see* Men
Malthus, T. R. 134
Maternal serum screening test 198
Medicines and pregnancy 202
Men
  and abortion 46, 55–8, 61–4, 65, 66–7, 68, 73, 74; broodiness 28; choice by 7; and contraception 35–42, 118; evasion of responsibility 13; and fertility 13, 154, impotence 156, 217; infertility 86, 156, 220; marginalisation 99; part in planning decisions 27–31; patriarchy 131–2,

135; reaction to pregnancy 45–7, 50–1; sperm tests 86; and sterilisation 75–6, 78–9
Menopause 156, 227, 229
Menstrual cycle 157–8, 159
   stressed 213
Menstrual extraction 192
Menstruation 112, 155, 157
Micro manipulation 225
Middle life pregnancies 211–12, 227–30
Mifepristone pill 193, 194
Miller, Warren B. 116–17
Mini-pill 161
Miscarriage, rate of 2
   see also Abortion
Moral aspects of fertility control 124–5, 207–10
   attitude to potential parents 10–11
Mosse, Julia 169
Motherhood as barrier to career 20
Multiple index method *see* Natural family planning
Multiple pregnancies 173, 222

Natural family planning 184–8
   effectiveness 186
Neonatology 124, 209
Neural tube defects, tests for 147
Norethisterone enanthate drug 176
Norplant, contraceptive device 146, 177–8

Occlusive devices 189
Oestrogen 158, 170
Oocytes 228
   donation 228, 229
Ovary, problems 214, 219, 221
Ovulation 155, 158, 159, 174, 218
   hindered by breast feeding 188; problems 214
Ovulation method of FP 185
Ovum *see* Egg

Parenthood, deferred 11–12
Parents
   preparation for pregnancy 200–10; questions for 138–40

Parents, adoptive *see* Adoptive parents
Patients
   calculated risk-takers 113–16; problematic 110–11; not respected 105–6
Patriarchy under attack 131–2, 135
Pelvic inflammatory disease (PID) 180, 183
Penis 157
Pergonal drug 173
Periods 158, 160
   irregular 218; and the pill 172, 175
Pill, contraceptive 36
   combined oral 170–3; failure rate 171; minipill 161; 'morning-after' pill 192; oral, avoidance pre- and during pregnancy 202; progestogen-only pill 174–5; use with barrier 173
Pituitary gland 156, 158
Polycystic ovary disease 214
Population explosion 5
'Pre-embryo' 169
Pregnancies
   affected by conditions 211; care during 199–203; ectopic 158, 175, 184, 190, 214; in middle-life 211–12, 227–30; and miscarriage 2; multi-problem case study 88–9; multiple 173, 222; one-person 30; planned or unplanned, proportion 5; reaction to 44; socially significant event 114; unplanned 9–10; unplanned and unwanted 43–4, 114–15; unwanted 133–4, 147, 193–5; wanted 195–200
Pregnancy tests 56
Pregnant women at risk 196
Premature babies 208–10
'Problem groups' and FP xi–xii
Procreation
   decision to bear children 15–16; urge to bear children 7, 16–18; reasons for 18–22
Professionals, health xiii, 103–8
   and unwanted pregnancies 133

Index

Progesterone 160, 161, 170
  injectable 175–7
Progesterone-only pill 174–5
  failure rate 174
Prostaglandin 194, 195
Psychiatrists 93–4
Puberty, age falling in girls 211

Radiotherapy and pregnancy 204
'Rational decision' on family planning 1–8
Relaxation recommended 213
Reproductive system 153–64
Retraint, alleged virtues of 11–12
Rhythm method, outmoded term 163
Risk-taking 118–19, 122–3, 149, 204, 235
RU 486 *see* Mifepristone
Rubella (German measles) 203

San Francisco Bay study of women 119–20
Sauer, M. V. 228
Sawhill, Isobel 146–7
Screening, pre-natal 147–8, 195–9
  see also Ultrasound
Services on offer, for FP 53
Sex
  a private event 114; unprotected 36–7
Sex education xi, 5, 106–7; changing 124, 135–6
Smoking
  and the pill 171, 172, 174; and pregnancy 201, 202
Special Baby Unit, John Radcliffe Hospital, Oxford 208
Sperm
  availability 159; count alleged to be lower 211; deficiency 221; and fertilisation 160, 164; male and female, separated 207; production 154, 156–7; quality 216–17; testing 86, 218–19, 220; and vasectomy 190
Sperm banks 225, 226
  donors 93, 226

Spermicides 178, 179, 180
  and condoms 181
Spina bifida, tests for 198, 200
Spinnbarkeit test 162
Sponge, contraceptive 181
Statistics 105
Sterilisation and men *see* Vasectomy
Sterilisation and women 76–8, 189–90
  case studies 76, 77–8; reversal 190;
  and Marie Stopes 133
Stillbirths 91–2
Stopes, Marie 132–3
Stress
  and infertility 87; during pregnancy 201
Stress cycles 213
Surrogate motherhood 5
Sympto-thermal method *see* Natural family planning

Temperature charts 86–7, 161–2
  Basal Body Temperature Charts (BBT) in FP 184, 218
Termination *see* Abortion
Testosterone 156
Thistle, Dr Jill 209
Toxoplasmosis 203–4
Triple-plus Test (Leeds Test) 198–9
Triple Test (Barts Test) 198
Trussell, Professor 212

Ultrasound scanning, pregnancy 197, 200, 219
Uncertainty factor 84
Unmarried women, refusal to treat 226
Urban Institute, Washington 147
Uterus 158, 159
  problems 215, 219

Vaccination
  before conception 203; against pregnancy 177
Vaginal ring 178
Vaginismus 216
Vasectomy 75, 78–9, 105, 190–1
Vault cap 178, 179

Vimule cap 179
Virginity 136
Visionary view of family creation 22–3

Weight control, during pregnancy 201
Wilson, Dr 212
Winston, Prof. 206–7, 221, 224, 228–9
Women
   biological complexity 112–13; conspiracy with doctors 131–2, 134–5; and contraception 35–42; decision-making freedom 134; fertility 27–31, 154; periods of transition 116–17; preference not to lie 40; and pregnancy 43–52; responsibility too much 7; view of vasectomy 79; work and change of balance 27

Young people, and decision on contraception 165–7